POCKET GUIDE TO
MIDWIFERY
CARE

AVIVA JILL ROMM

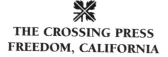

**THE CROSSING PRESS
FREEDOM, CALIFORNIA**

For information on bulk purchases or group discounts for this and
other Crossing Press titles, please contact our Special Sales
Manager at 800-777-1048 x214.

Visit our Web site on the Internet: www.crossingpress.com

Library of Congress Cataloging-in-Publication Data

Romm, Aviva Jill.
    Pocket guide to midwifery / by Aviva Jill Romm.
        p. cm.
    Includes bibliographical references.
    ISBN 0-89594-855-9
    1. Midwifery. 2. Midwives. I. Title.
RG950.R656   1998
618.2--dc21   98-10584
                                                                        CIP

Contents

Midwifery Care and Safety

A pregnant woman, protective of her child's well-being, is naturally going to wonder whether working with midwives will offer her the same level of safety for prenatal care and birth that she might expect from an obstetrician.

Fortunately, this question is also being asked by researchers, physicians, and midwives worldwide and there is a wealth of statistical evidence to help us sort through this safety question. While no method of care can guarantee specific outcomes in childbearing, statistical evidence based on numerous studies of midwifery care and out-of-hospital birth sites, including freestanding birthing centers and domiciliary sites (home), is exceptionally encouraging about the increased safety of childbearing when care is provided by a midwife, and especially by a midwife providing out-of-hospital care. In general, midwifery care has been shown to improve the general outcome with women and babies from a large variety of socioeconomic backgrounds, and to reduce difficult outcomes even in situations that are moderately high-risk. The World Health Organization (WHO), which has closely evaluated the safety of midwifery care, has recommended midwives as the ideal care providers for childbearing women worldwide.

The perinatal mortality rate (fetal and infant death rates from 20 weeks' gestation through the 28th day of life) is used as the statistic most directly relevant to the prenatal and birth period. In the United States approximately 70 percent of all infant deaths occur in the first 28 days after birth, and most of these deaths are related to events that occurred at birth, and also what occurred during the pregnancy (Wagner, 1988). Maternal morbidity (infection) and mortality are also

5

measured. These statistics will appear as numbers per thousand, that is 2 deaths per thousand births, or 10 deaths per thousand births. The higher the mortality rates, the poorer the outcomes being reflected. Many factors can influence morbidity and mortality rates, including maternal nutrition, hygiene, whether the mother smokes, prematurity, even place of birth. Whenever possible, studies are carried out in such a way so that the groups being compared have as many similar characteristics as possible, and that all things being relatively equal, a clear picture can emerge. For example, one cannot reasonably and fairly compare outcomes from homebirths and hospital births if all of the women who gave birth in the hospital were heavy smokers and all of the women who gave birth at home were non-smokers. The fact that smokers already have a higher risk of birth-related problems would make the study unreliable.

OBSTETRICIANS OR MIDWIVES, DOES IT MATTER?

It cannot be overstated that obstetrical care is an essential option for women with high-risk pregnancies, and for obstetrical emergencies. Yet in the United States, where 96 percent of babies are born in the hospital with obstetricians in attendance, the international infant mortality ranking is 23rd from the top, meaning that 22 countries have better infant mortality statistics than the United States. This is in stark contrast to births in the Netherlands where midwives deliver 50 percent of the babies, and Sweden where midwives deliver nearly 100 percent of the babies. These countries have infant mortality rankings of fourth and seventh respectively (World Population Data Sheet, 1988 Population Reference Bureau, Inc., Washington D.C.).

In every European country there is a large group of practicing midwives which far outweighs the number of obstetricians, and in each of these countries it is the midwives who provide primary health care to most healthy pregnant women (Wagner, 1988). In 1985, 36.6 percent of all Dutch babies were born at home, attended by direct-entry midwives (see Chapter 2 for an explanation of the different types of midwives), and the infant mortality rate was 1.9 per thousand (*British Journal of Obstetrics and Gynecology*, 1989). Repeated studies conducted by the British Government (1937, 1958, 1954–64, and 1970) further validate the safety of midwifery care; every study, including long-term studies, consistently demonstrated that midwifery (and homebirth) were safer for all but high-risk mothers and babies (Tew, 1990).

Why is it that we have come to assume that midwifery care is inferior to obstetric care? Perhaps it is because in the United States we have come to view childbirth as an inherently high-risk condition—a disease process—that requires medical supervision and intervention. In Europe, where the overall infant mortality rate is significantly lower than in the Unites States, "an important attitudinal difference accompanies the statistical difference. Europeans consider birth to be a normal event, and midwives deliver the majority of babies. Many European midwives work without physician supervision and are not required to study nursing as a prerequisite to midwifery training. Decades of misinformation, on the other hand, have taught women in the United States that birth is a dangerous and pathological event, requiring medical care by specialists. Obstetricians far outnumber midwives in our country and the excellent statistics of the midwives are a well-kept secret." (Suarez, 1993). A study done by the British Department of Health from 1970–72 found that even though midwives attended significantly more births in England than did obstetricians during those years, midwives were considered "responsible" for only 2 percent of the preventable maternal deaths. Compare this to hospital obstetrical staffs to which were attributed 67 percent of maternal deaths (Department of Health and Social Security, H.M.S.O., 1975). Clearly it is time to reevaluate our attitudes toward birth and midwifery care.

MORE STATISTICS

The things that count cannot be counted.

—unknown

Statistics supportive of midwifery care have come from studies conducted and recorded since as early as 1937 and have been done by independent researchers, as well as medical and governmental institutions, which do not necessarily benefit from results that support midwifery and homebirth. Even the American College of Obstetricians and Gynecologists, which states that the hospital is the safest place for all women to give birth, has not yielded a single published paper, scientific study, or analysis that clearly supports this assertion.

"Numerous studies have shown that maternity care provided by nurse-midwives *and other midwives* [my italics] in hospitals, birth centers, and homebirths result in birth-weights, infant mortality rates, and other health indicators similar to, or better than, those obtained by specialists in acute medical settings" (Women's Institute for Childbearing Policy, 1994). Dr. Enkin and his colleagues who compiled the longitudinal Oxford Database of Perinatal Trials, concluded that "...it is inherently unwise, and perhaps unsafe, for women with normal pregnancies to be cared for by obstetric specialists...Midwives and general practitioners, on the other hand, are primarily oriented to the care of women with normal pregnancies, and are likely to have more detailed knowledge of the particular circumstances of individual women. The care that they give to the majority of women whose pregnancies are not affected by any major illness or serious complication will often be more responsive to their needs than that given by specialist obstetricians" (Enkin, 1989). A study of 3,257 out-of-hospital births in Arizona, attended by lay midwives between 1978 and 1985 yielded a perinatal mortality rate of 2.2 per thousand (Sullivan and Wertz, 1988), in comparison with a national rate of 9.7 per thousand (Myron E. Wegman, *Annual Summary of Vital Statistics*–1990, 88 Pedatrics 1081, 1091 (1991), in Suarez, p. 338).

According to Dr. Charles Mahan, the Florida Deputy Secretary for Health, "If we are to make real progress in providing primary and preventative care and in reducing infant mortality rates, we must broaden our provider base by encouraging the growth of midwifery" (*Associated Press*, October, 1993).

Midwifery Care Provides More than Safety

It has been well-documented that during labor, the support and companionship of another woman can greatly reduce a woman's perception of discomfort, as well as the duration of labor and the incidence of complications. Midwives provide the mother with ongoing contact and support—physically and emotionally—during labor.

The success of midwifery care is self-evident when one looks at a randomized control trial done in 1988 (Women's

Institute for Childbearing Policy, 1994) which found that women working with midwives had an easier transition to motherhood than those working with obstetricians. This is because midwifery clients gain confidence in their abilities to parent, and have an increased sense of self-esteem. These qualities may reduce the incidence of psychological dysfunction in the family unit beyond the immediate childbearing experience, as well as reduce the incidence and severity of postpartum depression, a condition that can have far-reaching implications in the life of mother, child, and family.

Rates of breastfeeding are also higher among women who have used midwives for their care. Early postpartum breastfeeding is significantly higher among midwifery clients than among the general population, ranging from 78 to 99 percent of women who are able to breastfeed right after birth. In comparison, the rate of early postpartum breastfeeding for the general public in 1988 was 54 percent, and about half that for low-income and black mothers (United States Department of Health and Human Services, 1991).

Dr. J. G. Kloosterman, professor of Obstetrics and Gynecology at the University of Amsterdam and Director of the Midwives Academy in Holland from 1947 to 1957, has stated that under midwifery care only three to five percent of all healthy mothers would require the care of a physician at the time of birth, and if physicians were only consulted in three to five percent of cases the infant mortality rate would drop to between one and four per thousand (Suarez, 1993).

IS OBSTETRICS SAFEST?

When we begin to look at childbearing as an inherently natural, non-medical event, it becomes clear that midwives, trained to support women through this process and to deal with the variations of this process that naturally arise, are the best prepared to preserve the integrity of the birth process and of the women giving birth. And while obstetrics likes to take credit for reduced infant and maternal morbidity and mortality rates over the past century, "improved nutrition, sanitation, and other public health measures together with the increasing availability of effective contraception and a higher standard of living for women and infants have resulted in significant gains in basic health indicators (Thiery and Derom 1986; Shearer 1993; as in Women's Institute for Childbearing, 1994, p. 27).

Obstetrics cannot improve upon nature, yet this in some ways seems to be the intrinsic goal of this medical specialty. Some obstetricians see surgical delivery as an improvement over vaginal birth. If a vaginal birth is to occur, they feel that women must be protected from what obstetrics sees as irreparable and lifelong damage to the pelvic floor muscles as a result of the natural stretching of the vaginal tissues and musculature during birth. Hence we see an episiotomy rate of over 95 percent in many obstetric practices.

Dr. Kloosterman states, "By no means have we been able to improve spontaneous labor in healthy women. Spontaneous and normal labor is a process, marked by a series of events so perfectly attuned to one another that any interference only deflects them from their optimum course" (Kloosterman, J. G., *Why Midwifery?*, *The Practicing Midwife*, Spring, 1985).

Modern obstetrics, by its very interference in the birth process has accomplished less by trying to do more. Dr. Marsden Wagner, former Director of the World Health Organization's European Regional Office, remarked at an international medical conference that hospital births "endanger mothers and babies—primarily because of the impersonal procedures and overuse of technology and drugs" (Suarez, 1993). And the list of interventions is steadily increasing in the United States. Between 1984 and 1987 the following increases were shown: use of diagnostic ultrasound went up by 350 percent; use of fetal monitoring increased by 427 percent; manually assisted delivery increased 300 percent; vacuum extraction went up 132 percent; artificial rupture of membranes increased by 107 percent; medical labor induction increased 162 percent; repair of lacerations increased 39 percent; and cesarean sections increased 16 percent (Kozak as quoted in Suarez, 1993, p. 345).

Every intervention in the birth process is likely to disrupt the outcome of the entire process. Each interference can create another problem that is more complicated. For example, the use of external fetal monitoring (EFM) in labor causes women to be in a supine position, potentially reducing blood flow to the baby, thus creating a ripe environment for fetal distress. EFM, one of the apparently more benign medical interventions used in childbearing, has been associated with a higher percentage of cesarean sections in spite of there being no statistical improvement in outcome (Mold and Stein 1986; Wagner 1988; Fraser 1983; Brody and Thompson 1981; as in Women's Institute for Childbearing Policy 1994, p. 34). Variations in the heart rate as a result of the supine position leads to the use of an internal fetal monitor—an electrode literally screwed into the baby's scalp—increasing the likelihood of infection for the mother and child, and ensuring that the mother will now certainly be immobile for the rest of her labor, as it is extremely difficult to move around with wires extending from the vaginal canal, one of which is attached to the baby's head! Immobility in labor reduces the effectiveness of uterine contractions, reduces the mother's comfort and sense of control (relegates her to a "patient"), and further increases the likelihood of fetal distress. Reduced uterine effectiveness often leads to augmentation of the labor with pitocin, and this usually, but not always, leads to the mother wanting pain medication. The pitocin itself may have a derogatory effect on the baby's health and any pain medication given to a pregnant woman is known to cross the placenta and reach the baby. A well-controlled study done by an obstetrician at the University of Mississippi revealed that one out of every four infants whose mothers had received "only 50 milligrams of meperidine (Demerol) within one to three hours before delivery required resuscitation at birth" (Suarez, 1993). These combined factors increase the likelihood of fetal distress, the necessity of a cesarean section for the delivery of the child, or the increased likelihood of breathing difficulties that arise from central nervous system depression caused by the pain medications should be born vaginally. I will not immediately go into the risks of cesareans, but there are many. The Oxford researchers mentioned earlier in this chapter also concluded that "hospitals and staff members who oversee births—primarily doctors and nurses—routinely employ some methods of care that ultimately not only offer little benefit to mother or infant but might actually be dangerous to them" (Ubell, 1993). According to these researchers, when normal pregnancy is treated like a disease, it has a very poor outcome (Ubell 1993; Suarez 1993). Furthermore, new techniques are regularly being adopted, though they may not be thoroughly evaluated for long-term safety. Sophisticated diagnostic techniques may lead to interventions that are not proven to be remedial (Tew, 1985).

In addition to the increased risk of physical harm resulting from routine medical interventions, "it is possible that the unfamiliar setting and the presence of unfamiliar personnel, the limited presence and role of family members, and the restricted freedom of movement of the laboring woman may all create an atmosphere that undermines self-confidence and encourages passivity on the part of the laboring woman, diminishing her ability to deliver spontaneously" (Durand, 1992).

CESAREAN SECTIONS

Cesarean sections, episiotomy, repair of obstetric lacerations, and artificial rupture of membranes accounted for 18 percent of all surgical procedures that were done in hospitals in 1990 (National Center for Health Statistic Surveys, United States Department of Health and Human Services, Discharge Survey, Annual Summary, 1990). Cesarean section is the most frequently performed surgery in the United States, and the most frequently performed unnecessary surgery. It is estimated that 473,000 unnecessary cesareans were done in the United States in 1991 alone. More than two dozen women are estimated to have died as a result of this procedure during that year. Current national statistics reveal a cesarean section rate that is alarming: nearly one in four women having a baby will undergo a cesarean.

The risks to the woman undergoing the cesarean are significant, and cesareans are only warranted in a very small percentage of cases. Increased risks include uterine infection, bladder infection, increased risk of abnormal blood-clotting and therefore dangerous emboli, injury to the surrounding organs, infertility, adverse psychological response, and death. Approximately 4.2 to 18.9 percent of women who have a cesarean will experience an immediate complication of surgery (Gabay and Wolfe, 1994).

Also, one of eight babies born by cesarean section will develop respiratory distress syndrome (RDS) due to errors in the timing of the procedure—that is surgery being done electively before the baby's lungs are fully mature (Suarez 1993)—and possibly due to a lack of the physiological processes of vaginal birth which prepare a neonate's lungs for breathing. RDS can lead to neonatal death, and it is also a major factor associated with Sudden Infant Death Syndrome (SIDS).

Clearly, under specific circumstances, obstetric technologies outweigh the risks associated with them. However, when access to technology is widely available these technologies become broadly applied in a population where their use is not warranted. It is when technologies are applied in this way that they are associated with the poorest outcomes. Research directed toward the "development of ever more sophisticated technology and away from establishing the conditions in which birth is safest...has directed the education of not only obstetricians, but also of midwives and general practitioners towards mastering the skills of high technology and away from the skills of low-technology midwifery, which results show to be the safest for the great majority of births" (Tew, 1985). Statistical analysis of thousands of births in Holland showed that the perinatal mortality rate was significantly lower when women were under the care of midwives rather than obstetricians as the primary caregivers (Tew, Marjorie, and SMI

Damastra-Wijmenga, Safest Birth Attendants: Recent Dutch Evidence. Midwifery, 1991, 7:55–63).

Cesarean Section Rates

Country	Number of Cesarean Sections per 100 Births
Czechoslovakia	7
Japan	7
Hungary	10
Netherlands	10
England and Wales (U.K.)	10
New Zealand	10
Switzerland	11
Norway	12
Spain	12
Sweden	12
Greece	13
Portugal	13
Italy	13
Denmark	13
Scotland	14
Bavaria	15
Australia	16
Canada	19
United States	23
Puerto Rico	29
Brazil	32

Francis C. Notzon, *International Differences in the Use of Obstetric Interventions*, 263 Journal of the American Medical Association 3286, 3287 (1990).

The countries that utilize midwives as the primary caregivers for childbearing women have not only the lowest perinatal mortality rates, but the lowest cesarean section rates. "Countries with some of the lowest perinatal mortality rates in the world have cesarean section rates of less than 10 percent. There is no justification for any region to have a rate higher than 10 to 15 percent" (Wagner, 1988).

Compare this to the cesarean section rate of nearly 25 percent in the United States. This is even higher in some communities: 16 hospitals in the United States had cesarean section rates of higher than 45 percent or more (Gabay and Wolfe 1994) and at the Lakota reservation in South Dakota in 1990, the cesarean section rate was 66 percent (Leonard Littlefinger, director of BIA hospital, personal communication, 1989). According to studies using matched or adjusted cohorts—meaning groups that have characteristics closely resembling each other—"U.S. women beginning labor with midwives and/or in out-of-hospital settings have attained cesarean section rates that are considerably lower than similar women using prevailing forms of care—physicians in hospitals. This cesarean reduction involved no compromise in morbidity and mortality outcome measures. Moreover, groups of women at elevated risk for adverse perinatal outcomes have attained excellent outcomes and cesarean rates well below the general population rate with these care arrangements" (Sakala 1993).

Midwifery care also reduces the incidence of prematurity by providing excellent social support, attention to nutrition, and attention to lifestyle. Education aimed at reducing significant risk factors such as drug use, smoking, and infection is also a part of midwifery care. The greatest single factor leading to perinatal mortality is premature birth. Babies weighing 2.5 kilograms (5.5 pounds) or less account for six percent of live births and two-thirds of all perinatal deaths.

Safety and the Law
"By their philosophy and training, midwives are the most appropriate medical care providers to confront the growing

crisis in high-risk infants, and to help provide the preventive care so desperately needed" (Midwives' Alliance of New York, 1990). While conventional maternity services have "regularly been found to be impersonal, fragmented, inconvenient, and neither community-oriented nor culturally appropriate" (Women's Institute for Childbearing Policy 1994), midwifery care is highly personal, integrated into the context of a woman's life, and community and culturally sensitive. Legalizing the status of midwives within the realm of childbearing professionals would allow for greater accessibility and convenience.

ECONOMIC VALUE OF MIDWIFERY CARE

Midwifery care is practical on economic grounds as well as for reasons of safety. According to Gabay and Wolfe (1994), the unnecessary cesareans done in 1991 (of which 50 percent were deemed unnecessary) cost the American public more than $1.3 billion. According to Dr. Frank Oski, M.D., professor and Director of the Department of Pediatrics, Johns Hopkins University School of Medicine, "From $13 to $20 billion a year could be saved in health care costs by developing a network of midwifery care providers, demedicalizing childbirth, and encouraging breastfeeding." [When] "every country in Europe with perinatal and infant mortality rates lower than the U.S. uses midwives as the principal birth attendant for at least 70 percent of all births" it really ought to make us sit up and rethink some of our ideas (Wagner quoted in Report of the New York State Department of Health Ad Hoc Advisory Committee on the Education and Recruitment of Midwives, June 1988).

HOMEBIRTH WITH MIDWIVES: RADICAL OR REASONABLE?

While the advantages of homebirth are discussed later, here I document evidence that illustrates the safety of homebirth with a midwife over conventional medical care in a hospital setting. In an article in *Nursing Times* (November 20, 1985) Marjorie Tew states that, "When the results of aggregated experience are impartially analyzed, they consistently show that birth is in fact safer when the level of intervention is low. The overall perinatal mortality rate is *always* [my italics] found to be higher in hospitals than at home with normal midwifery care." When this type of study is extended to high-risk mothers, the results are that unpredicted risks are still considerably higher in hospitals than at home.

Interventions in childbearing increase the rates of complications and reduce the safety of the experience for women and children. The safety of homebirth with a midwife is directly related to the fact that midwives are trained not interfere with the birth process unless it is necessary to do so. Midwives are not inherently opposed to interventions, but midwifery supports a philosophy of appropriate technology, that is, the judicious use of medical procedures when relevant, but not routinely.

In the Farm Study, homebirths attended by lay midwives appear to have been accomplished with safety comparable to that of conventional births, with a significantly reduced incidence of births that required operative assistance (Duran). In Kentucky, a study of planned versus unplanned homebirths (1981 to 1983) found that for 214 planned midwife-attended homebirths there were no neonatal deaths (*Journal of the American Medical Association*, 1985, Volume 253). Albers and Katz, in an article for the

Journal of Nurse-Midwifery concluded based upon a review of the literature, that "nontraditional birth settings present advantages for low-risk women as compared with traditional hospital settings: lower costs for maternity care, and lower use of childbirth procedures, without significant differences in perinatal mortality" (Albers and Katz 1991).

From a Norwegian study (Olsen 1994): "all statistical comparisons relevant to Nordic women today show that for healthy pregnant women it is at least as safe to give birth at home—and perhaps even safer." Furthermore, many randomized clinical trials consistently show that several of the elements which characterize homebirths make the births proceed much easier. It should be clearly understood that the positive statistical outcomes in Europe and other countries utilizing midwifery care as the primary care for pregnant women are based on the work of *non-nurse* midwives, known in the United States as direct-entry midwives.

It is not well-known to the American public that there are several thousand direct-entry midwives in the United States, attending homebirths and running clinics and birthing centers. Despite the fact that a growing base of research demonstrates that direct-entry midwifery care is equally effective to nurse-midwifery care, most research in the U.S. has been funded by institutions that support institutionalized midwifery training. The literature shows that homebirths attended by direct-entry midwives with low-to-moderate-risk women are at least as safe as hospital births attended by either physicians or nurse-midwives (Haffner-Eaton and Pearce 1994). Births attended by midwives out of hospital had a significantly lower risk for low birthweight than those attended in hospitals by certified nurse-midwives (Janssen, Holt, and Myers 1994).

The fact that direct-entry midwives, unlike nurse-midwives, practice without the limitations imposed by a supervisory obstetrician is significant in that midwives' intervention rates go up when under the control of obstetricians' protocols and policies, and intervention rates are lower when midwives practice independently (Goer 1995). Midwifery can, and should be, an autonomous profession. The cooperation of the medical community, rather than supervision or control, only increases the safety and positive outcomes for families choosing to work with independent midwives and to have their babies at home.

Independent midwives also present cost savings for parents. Normal vaginal delivery with an obstetrician in a hospital costs as much as $5000 to $8000, with an additional $2000 on average for a cesarean section. The average cost of midwifery care in the United States is approximately $1500, with prices varying slightly according to the communities served. To initiate care with an obstetrician it is common to have to pay a sum as large as $1500 up front, whereas with a midwife, payment is usually flexible and divided over the course of care.

It is my hope that by now your curiosity is piqued about midwifery care. Read on and discover who midwives are, and what they do.

Different Types of Midwives

The simplest definition of midwifery is "with woman," but truly, midwifery means different things to different people. For many, the Midwifery Model is an attitude about women and how pregnancy and birth occur, and a view that pregnancy and birth are normal events until proven otherwise. It is an attitude of giving and sharing information, of empowerment, and of respecting the right of a woman and her family to determine their own care.

from FAQ sheet, MANA, Thursday, June 20, 1996

MIDWIFE MEANS "WITH WOMAN"

Many languages have a term to describe the women who attend other women in childbirth: in Spanish it is *Comadrona*, the one who is with woman, also meaning a woman friend; in French it is *Sage Femme*, wise woman; in Danish it is *Jordemoder*—Earth Mother; in Hawaiian it is *Pale Keiki* or protector of the child; and in KiSwahili it is *Mkunga*, which means confidential advisor.

The history and traditions of midwifery vary from culture to culture, but one thing is certain: historically midwives have had an instrumental role as not only the women who "catch the babies," but as personal health care advisors and intimate confidantes to the personal and sexual lives of the women in their communities at their various stages of sexual development, often serving families "from the cradle to the grave." Midwives were also the community herbalists, or family doctors as we would now call them, being referred to in times of illness that went beyond the often formidable level of knowledge of the average house-holding woman.

A BIT OF BACKGROUND

In the United States midwifery has existed through the continuous presence of community-based midwives, such as the pioneer midwives, immigrant midwives, and the plantation midwives, who were often slaves, the Grand midwives, and now through the modern midwifery community—the direct-entry midwives of today. It is true that many midwives well into the early part of this century were uneducated by formal standards, yet early statistics reveal that these women were demonstrating birth outcomes far superior to those of the regular doctors of their day. In 1911, a study done by Johns Hopkins University School of Medicine stated that by the time of graduation most medical students had never delivered a baby, and that a quarter of medical school graduates were not competent to practice obstetrics. In February of 1913 the *American Journal of Public Health* reported that midwives had much better outcomes than did their physician contemporaries, and research conducted from 1930 to 1932 by the New York Academy of Medicine revealed that the death rate of childbearing women was higher when births were attended by doctors than by midwives. It is important to realize that the approach of midwives was, and continues to be, one of trusting nature to take its course, and realizing that this happens best when the process is not interfered with. This is very different from medical treatment of the 18th through early 20th centuries when the use of mercury, bloodletting, and the frequent application of forceps were in vogue.

THE CONTEMPORARY MIDWIFE

By 1930 the number of births attended by midwives in the United States was a mere 15 percent (it had been about 50 percent at the turn of the century, and higher prior to that). Due to lack of an organized professional base, generally low levels of formalized education, and the isolation of midwives from one community to the next, it was relatively easy for the medical profession to publicly undermine the credibility of midwives, and due to their inability to counter public attack, the number of midwives declined. However, in 1925, nurse-midwifery as a formal profession was introduced here by way of Great Britain, and a resurgence in midwifery slowly began.

The Frontier Nursing Service, a practice of community nurses in Kentucky, with the desire to improve the health of rural and poor Appalachian women, began to recruit nurses and send them to England for midwifery training. These women then attended childbirths in Appalachia, often riding on horseback to women's homes at all hours of the day and night. Their commitment to childbearing women in this region resulted in mortality statistics lower than those for the rest of the state of Kentucky, and in the United States as a whole. By the beginning of World War II, the Frontier Nursing Service was training its own midwives. Meanwhile, in New York City, nurse-midwives were also beginning to set up training programs to serve poor women, and by 1955 the American College of Nurse-Midwives (ACNM) was established as the professional organization for nurse-midwives, though there were still very few at the time. It wasn't until the 1970s that the numbers of midwives began to grow, and until the 1980s that middle- and upper-class women began to use nurse-midwifery care regularly. However, this care was influenced and circumscribed by the medical traditions of the day, and even now, nurse-midwives in hospitals, though bringing great improvement to hospital birthing, are limited by hospital policy and the protocols of overseeing obstetricians.

During the 1970s, many women were still strapped down for birth—with feet in stirrups, flat on their backs—after having been given a pubic shave and an enema, and separated from their loved ones and all that was familiar. At this time small groups of women around the Unites States began to question what they perceived as an overly medicalized and anti-woman approach to childbirth. Supported by the growing women's movement, as well as by a few mavericks in the field of obstetrics such as Grantly Dick-Read and Frederick Leboyer, women began to demand greater choice and freedom in the hospitals. A small but powerful number of women even began to take childbirth back into their own hands, having homebirths and learning to become midwives. They did this through a variety of routes, either simply by being there for each other, or through self-study, study groups, and study with supportive doctors, nurse-midwives, and other health care professionals. This movement of women has grown into the formal profession of direct-entry midwifery in the United States and saw the birth, in 1983, of a professional organization for the support of direct entry-midwifery, the Midwives Alliance of North America (MANA). MANA is one of the two largest midwifery organizations (along with the ACNM) in the United States and has an international membership that includes direct-entry midwives, certified professional midwives, certified nurse-midwives, medical doctors, and non-midwife members such as childbirth educators and other advocates of midwifery and the rights of childbearing women.

Direct-entry midwives believe that childbearing women should have access to a wide variety of knowledge-able care providers so that they might choose the type of care and care provider that best suits their needs. In this light, the remainder of this book is devoted to providing you with greater insight into midwifery care, so that you may have a fuller range of options from which to choose.

TYPES OF MIDWIVES

Midwives from all backgrounds come to their work with a great love and respect for women, babies, and children, as well as respecting the philosophy that birth is a natural process that happens best when women are respected, treat-ed well, nurtured and supported, but not interfered with.

Unfortunately the professions of midwifery and certi-fied nurse-midwifery are burdened with politics, particular-ly pressures being placed on both groups by obstetricians, hospitals, insurance agencies, and health maintenance com-panies. In addition, the ACNM has targeted non-nurse midwives as competition, and has recently been using its allegiance with obstetrics and universities to denounce the importance and safety of direct-entry midwifery. This is so, even in spite of the fact that many certified nurse-midwives enjoy close professional relationships with direct-entry midwives, and many respect the importance of having both CNMs and DEMs available. Nonetheless, this tension has often served to divide what could be one tremendous effort to support women, babies, and families, into disparate groups often working at odds with each other. And as is the case in many groups with opposing factions, the greater vision often gets lost in the struggle. This book is a reminder of the importance of unity in diversity, with the greater goal of improving maternal and child wellness.

Direct-Entry Midwives

> *Care that is provided by another woman can be special. A midwife is a birthing woman's equal, not her authority. She is a confidante. She understands the importance of being respectful and gentle with another person's most intimate parts of herself. She knows that safety in childbirth is more a matter of prevention than treatment, of learning to listen closely, helping a woman have a healthy attitude, and promoting normalcy...She protects both the privacy of the woman and the integrity of the family.*
>
> —Elizabeth Davis, *Heart and Hands:*
> *A Midwife's Guide to Pregnancy and Birth*

There are estimated to be between 4,000 and 6,000 direct-entry midwives in the United States. Midwives are committed to providing the kind of care, knowledge, and skill that supports women in making the transition to motherhood with strength, health, joy, and a sense of personal empowerment for both the women and their families.

The term "direct-entry midwife" (DEM) is derived from the European model where midwives are trained in a program that does not require any nursing training or a nursing degree. In the United States direct-entry midwife broadly refers to any midwife who practices without prior nursing training, though some DEMs are nurses who prefer to enter midwifery directly rather than training as a nurse-midwife. Any midwife who is not a CNM may be considered a direct-entry midwife. Under the title of DEM comes a wide variety of midwives. Some may call themselves traditional midwives, independent midwives, community midwives, domiciliary midwives, or other names that reflect a bit of their philosophy or approach. Under this category also come direct-entry midwives who are Licensed Midwives and Certified Professional Midwives.

Midwives in Europe refer to what the DEMs in the U.S. practice as "core midwifery." What this means, or better yet reflects, is that midwives here are practicing midwifery that is not institutionally bound and dictated, but midwifery that is based on the core needs of the women giving birth. It is midwifery that retains what is important and fundamental to the preservation of healthy childbearing, including the integrity of the women birthing. Institutionalization tends to give rise to requirements that fit the purpose and longevity of the institution and may easily override the needs and concerns of those whom the institution ought to serve. In fact, the personal need of the mother to have a sense of empowerment or fulfillment in the pregnancy or birth process is often seen as a selfish emotional need on her part, rather than an integral factor for the health of the mother and her child. Self-esteem may actually be a key factor in healthy parenting and for healthy children. What we have seen in America is that women come to see themselves as subordinate to the institutions that they enlist for reproductive health care—the obstetricians and gynecologists, the hospitals, and the hospital staff. Truly, the institutions should be working for us, not the other way around. This is what core midwifery seeks to preserve—the centrality of the mother/baby/family in the process of childbearing.

Midwives generally possess a high level of academic knowledge and clinical skills, learned through a combination of formal study and apprenticeship or attendance at one of the several midwifery colleges in this country. Many women who come to midwifery as a profession have themselves given birth, and this imparts a unique level of empirical knowledge that can be gained in no other way.

In the apprenticeship model, midwives gain their clinical experience by attending prenatal examinations, births, and postpartum visits, etc., under the guidance of an experienced preceptor, usually another DEM. Some of this training may also be done with a certified nurse-midwife, an obstetrician, family physician, osteopath, or other practitioner skilled in caring for childbearing women. An apprenticeship generally lasts for several years, until both the student and mentor feel confident that the new midwife is prepared to serve as a primary practitioner or until the student meets certification or licensing criteria. Academic work may occur in the context of guided study with the preceptor, independent scholarship, attendance of courses at a university, through a reputable home-study course, or through a combination of these approaches.

DEMs may also gain midwifery training at one of the nearly dozen accredited midwifery programs or midwifery colleges, or at one of the accredited naturopathic schools in the United States offering midwifery training. These schools are independent institutions in states where direct-entry midwifery is legally recognized as a health care profession. The training is usually a three-year program that combines academic and clinical education, or a year or more of postgraduate training when done in conjunction with training as a naturopathic physician. More midwifery programs are expected to open in the next five years, and the Midwifery Education and Accreditation Council (MEAC), a sister organization to the Midwives Alliance of North

America, is overseeing many of these schools through accrediting according to Department of Education standards, while still honoring the validity of the various routes to midwifery training, including apprenticeship.

DEMs are skilled in the care of women in their reproductive years, capable of providing primary care throughout pregnancy, birth, the postpartum needs of the mother and baby, as well as in well-woman gynecology, such as breast-exam, gynecological exam and counseling, sexuality counseling, and family planning. DEMs are also well versed in the psycho-emotional needs of women in various stages of their reproductive years, and many DEMs work with teenagers and women in menopause, as well as providing a broad range of counseling to mothers.

Most DEMs attend childbirth at home, but in states where midwifery is legally recognized, midwives may work at or run birthing centers, or they may work in a medical office with obstetricians and nurse-midwives. DEMs may work alone, in practices with other DEMs, or in practice with nurse-midwives, naturopaths, or other practitioners. Midwives provide prenatal care in a variety of settings: at the midwife's home, at an office, at the home of the pregnant woman, or in a clinic. Postpartum visits are usually done both at the new mother's home in the days after the birth, and then back at the midwife's office several weeks after the birth for further follow-up. DEMs are trained to recognize, understand, and treat problems that may arise in the childbearing process, and learn to detect these early so that women can be referred to obstetricians when necessary.

The World Health Organizations definition of the midwife gives us the following guidelines:

She must be able to give the necessary supervision, care, and advice to women during pregnancy, labor, and the postpartum period, to conduct deliveries on her own responsibility and to care for the newborn and the infant. This care includes preventative measures, the detection of abnormal conditions in mother and child, the procurement of medical assistance and the execution of emergency measures in the absence of medical help. She has an important task in health counseling and education, not only for the woman, but also within the family and the community. The work should involve antenatal education and preparation for parenthood and extend to certain areas of gynecology, family planning and child care. She may practice in hospitals, clinics, health care units, domiciliary conditions or in any other service. (WHO, FICO, ICM Statement)

from FAQ sheet, MANA, October 6, 1995, off of America Online, Thursday, June 20, 1996

Grand Midwives

The term "grand midwife" refers to those women who have practiced midwifery since before 1965, or thereabouts. Prior to the term "grand midwife" (coined by members of the Midwives Alliance of North America in the 1980s), these women were usually called granny midwives. The name was changed to grand midwife to more accurately reflect the respect these women deserve for their seniority and wisdom. The history of the grand midwife, rich and inspiring, has been recorded in a few biographies, but many of the grand midwives have passed on from this world, taking their stories with them. These stories tell of the struggle of the poor, as these are the people who have often been served by these women, as well as of the varied cultures of people, as it is often ethnic communities who have maintained their grand midwife traditions the longest.

Midwives

This category refers to direct-entry midwives who are uncertified and unlicensed, which may be the case for a variety of reasons including lack of available certification/licensure in the midwife's community or state, political, philosophical, or religious views against certification and licensure, or lack or experience to qualify for available certification or licensure.

Due to political and legal attempts on the part of the medical community to minimize the number of midwives practicing legally in the United States, many midwives have practiced without any legal recognition, and though they may wish to be members of the legally recognized professional health community, no such vehicles exist for them. Some midwives may deliberately choose to maintain an unlicensed or uncertified status, even when such certification or licensing vehicles exist, in order to protect the rights of childbearing women to birth where, how, and with whom they choose. Religious midwives may choose to remain entirely autonomous, seeing God as their only authority, and decline to be certified or licensed.

Most midwives study through one of the various routes previously described, and bring to their clients great skill, conviction, autonomy, and support. Because uncertified/unlicensed midwives are completely independent, they are responsible to none but themselves and the families they serve. This has tremendous advantages for childbearing women today, because governing boards in the field of obstetrics, who often oversee midwives, tend to impose very narrow limitations on what is considered low-risk and therefore allowable in the realm of midwifery care, particularly for homebirth. Midwives who are certified or licensed may be limited in some areas of practice due to the constraints of their affiliation's regulations.

Midwives practicing in states where midwifery is illegal may have well-established support networks, knowledge of local hospitals, and relationships with local obstetricians and pediatricians that can afford one a sense of having access to such care should one want or need it. Unfortunately, the illegality of midwives often prohibits such relationships from developing, as doctors are fearful of personal liability and increasing malpractice insurance rates should they become involved with direct-entry midwives. In no state is access to medical care unavailable to women in need, and hospitals must accept women and babies requiring medical attention.

The primary disadvantage to working with an uncertified or unlicensed midwife is that you—as a woman seeking midwifery care—have no external verification other than references, of the credentials and qualifications of midwives you interview. As in all professions (including obstetrics) there are those who would exaggerate their skills or knowledge in order to build a business, and unfortunately, midwifery is not immune to this phenomenon. Also, though the apprenticeship model of education is a very successful model, without any guidelines, a less experienced or less-than-competent midwife can pass on to her students an education which is not thorough, resulting in poorly trained midwives. Bear in mind that certification and licensing of midwives is no more a guarantee of integrity in midwifery than is that of licensed doctors in medicine. There are numerous recorded cases of medical incompetence, iatrogenic (doctor-caused) complications, and a lack of integrity among licensed medical doctors and other health care professionals.

It becomes the responsibility and task of parents seeking midwifery care (or any other forms of health care) to be very clear in what their own expectations are in of midwife, and to be fastidious in their efforts to understand the philosophies, skills, and limitations of the midwife with whom they plan to work. See Chapter 5 "Choosing a Midwife," for further information.

Certified and Licensed Midwives

In some states midwives may be certified through the state midwifery organization or they may be certified or licensed though the state government. This provides parents with some knowledge of the standards for the qualifications of the midwives in their area, and also tends to increase a midwife's access to involvement in the medical community, facilitating medical back-up for clients and easing such concerns as how one would transport to the hospital from a homebirth if there is a problem. Certified and licensed midwives may also be free to carry and administer certain medications, to suture, and to use IVs however this is not always the case.

There are disadvantages to state licensing requirements and standards for midwifery practice. For example, some states require that a pregnant mother working with a midwife see an obstetrician for a specific number of visits prenatally. Some women wish not to do this, seeing it as an infringement on their right to privacy. This puts the midwife in a compromised position, as she may be empathetic to the mother's concerns, but she is bound by the terms of her license to require this of the mother. She may feel forced to terminate care with parents who refuse to see medical practitioners during pregnancy, leaving parents without the guidance they might desire from a midwife.

Similarly, certification and licensing requirements may prohibit midwives from serving women who fall into certain narrow risk categories. Another disadvantage to the licensing or certification requirements of certain states is that they do not accept the apprenticeship model as a valid educational route, and thus require three years of attendance at a formally approved midwifery college. Requirements for education at an institution can effectively prohibit the women who are best suited to midwifery from entering this profession.

The Certified Professional Midwife

In response to a growing crisis in maternity care in the United States, as well as elsewhere, the Midwives' Alliance of North America and the North American Registry of Midwives (NARM), the overseeing organization for certified professional midwives (CPMs), developed a certification program to provide standards for direct-entry midwifery care, and a method for verifying these standards. These standards, developed with the guidance of independent testing organizations, have been created by midwives for midwives. Those who choose to participate in this process and meet these standards are qualified to be known as Certified Professional Midwives.

Certified Professional Midwives uphold, promote, and practice the midwifery model of care which emphasizes guarding the physical, psychological, and social well-being of the mother throughout the childbearing cycle; providing the mother with individualized education, counseling, and prenatal care, continuous hands-on assistance during labor and delivery, and postpartum support; minimizing technological interventions; and identifying and referring women who require medical attention. CPMs gain their training through the routes previously described for DEMs and midwives in general, but after their training is complete they qualify to be a CPM through an extensive application process, a written examination, and a clinical examination referred to as a skills assessment (the testing process is monitored and evaluated by an independent psychometrics organization). There are also requirements for continuing education and a process of peer review. At the time of this writing there are approximately 300 CPMs practicing in the United States.

Many states that have midwifery licensure have adopted the NARM written examination as their licensing exam, and it is the hope of NARM that this certification process may become nationally, and perhaps internationally recognized as a standard for midwifery training and care.

There are many advantages to the CPM process, the primary one being that it is a standard set by midwives for midwives, rather than an externally and arbitrarily based set of guidelines. With a great deal of effort and time, midwives across the United States have contributed to the development of standards for education and practice that are rigorous enough to provide for excellent quality of care, yet sensitive enough to women to allow for flexibility in midwifery practice. The women becoming CPMs believe strongly that midwifery should be a completely independent profession, and are working hard to preserve the right to independent practice.

The primary motivation of women seeking to become CPMs is the desire to see midwifery care become a more widely available option for women from varying economic and social backgrounds. In addition, many midwives feel that they can provide more relaxed care when they themselves are not practicing outside of the law.

The Midwives' Alliance of North America acknowledges the importance of all midwives who—with or without formal credentials—are offering midwifery services to childbearing women. Certified Professional Midwives practice according to the MANA Standards and Guidelines for the Art and Practice of Midwifery, and in accordance with the MANA Statement of Values and Ethics. While the standards for the CPM are high, it can be achieved through a variety of modes including apprenticeship, independent scholarship, attendance at a midwifery school, or by becoming a CNM first.

The Midwives Alliance of North America recognizes that while formal validation of knowledge and skills can be useful measures of one's abilities and educational accomplishments and therefore supports the certification process for midwives, no exams and certification can assure quality of practice or accurately measure a midwife's experience or intuitive understanding of midwifery. They therefore also encourage midwives and parents to work together on the basis of informed consent, and for parents to choose the practitioner in their community that best serves their personal needs and expectations.

Certified Nurse-Midwives

Certified nurse-midwives are registered nurses who then gain advanced training in midwifery. This may be done with a certificate program after a two-year nursing degree with a bachelor's degree in either the arts or sciences, or as a master's degree program after a four-year nursing degree. The midwifery training is generally done at a college or university, with the midwife interning at a clinic, birthing center, or hospital; or it may be done through a home study course (through the Frontier School of Nursing program) with an internship that is supervised by a CNM in a hospital, birthing center, clinic, or homebirth practice. Many CNMs began their careers as labor and delivery nurses and some began as direct-entry midwives. At present it is estimated that there are about 4,500 certified nurse-midwives in the United States.

CNMs are legally able to attend births in a variety of settings including homebirths, but for this they require the back-up of an obstetrician, which may be hard to find. In addition, the costs of medical malpractice insurance for midwives combined with the scarcity of medical back-up make it difficult for CNMs to maintain private practices.

In direct competition with the growing numbers of direct-entry midwives and particularly in response to the certification of direct-entry midwives through the CPM process and the growing popularity of homebirth, the American College of Nurse-Midwives has instituted a non-nurse midwifery training program, whereby one, without prior experience in any health care profession and with the sole requirement of having a Bachelor of Arts degree in any subject, may attend a training program for one year and then be certified to practice midwifery and legally attend homebirths upon passing a midwifery examination. As of this writing, this program is only available at one university in New York state, and has only one graduate to date. This training is clearly inferior to the wealth of experience and knowledge brought to midwifery care by the certified professional midwife. In spite of this political move by the leadership of the ACNM, many CNMs are highly supportive of direct-entry midwifery, and a growing number of CNMs and DEMs (including CPMs) are working cooperatively in practices.

The Care Midwives Give

"The Midwifery Model of Care" is based on the fact that pregnancy and birth are normal life events. The Midwifery Model of Care includes: tending to the physical, psychological, and social well-being of the mother with individualized education, counseling, and prenatal care, continuous hands-on assistance during labor and birth, and postpartum support; minimizing technological interventions; and identifying and referring women who require medical attention. The application of this woman-centered model has been proven to reduce the incidence of birth injury, trauma, and cesarean section.

—modified from MANA News, July, 1996

MOTHER AND BABY ARE CENTRAL FOCUS OF CARE

Midwifery is an art and science that is centered on the individual rather than the institution. A midwife makes it the central task of her practice to get to know the women with whom she works. This allows her a level of intimacy that enables her to provide care that is attentive to the physical needs of the mother and baby, as well as to the emotional, psychological, and spiritual needs of the mother, baby, and family. This sensitivity can also be found in a midwife's care of women at other stages in their life, such as puberty and menopause. To this relationship with women and families she brings her extensive knowledge base and practical experience, recognizing that a healthy mother and baby—on all levels—is her primary goal. This approach, which has come to be referred to as "The Midwifery Model of Care," is the bedrock of midwifery practice.

This chapter will take you, step by step, through the care you might expect to receive from a midwife from before conception to beyond the birth of your child. Midwifery practices will vary, as each midwife's personality, background, place of practice, and beliefs influence her approach.

Guiding Principles of Midwifery Practice

The midwife provides care according to the following principles:

- Midwives work in partnership with women and their chosen support community throughout the care-giving relationship.
- Midwives respect the dignity, rights and the ability of the women they serve to act responsibly throughout the care-giving relationship.
- Midwives work as autonomous practitioners, collaborating with other health and social service providers when necessary.
- Midwives understand that physical, emotional, psycho-social and spiritual factors synergistically comprise the health of individuals and affect the childbearing process.
- Midwives understand that female physiology and childbearing are normal processes, and work to optimize the well-being of mothers and their developing babies as the foundation of care-giving.
- Midwives understand that the childbearing experience is primarily a personal, social, and community event.
- Midwives recognize that a woman is the only direct care provider for herself and her unborn baby; thus the most important determinant of a healthy pregnancy is the mother herself.
- Midwives recognize the empowerment inherent in the childbearing experience and strive to support women to make informed choices and take responsibility for their own well-being.

- Midwives strive to ensure vaginal birth and provide guidance and support when appropriate to facilitate the spontaneous processes of pregnancy, labor, and birth, utilizing medical intervention only as necessary.
- Midwives synthesize clinical observations, theoretical knowledge, intuitive assessment and spiritual awareness as components of a competent decision-making process.
- Midwives value continuity of care throughout the childbearing cycle and strive to maintain continuous care within realistic limits.
- Midwives understand that the parameters of "normal" vary widely and recognize that each pregnancy and birth are unique.

MANA Core Competencies: Guiding Principles of Practice

PRENATAL CARE

Women may choose to begin a relationship with a midwife at any point in the pregnancy, or even before pregnancy. Most midwives will speak with you by telephone to set up an initial consultation, which consists of a visit to her office that provides an opportunity for you to meet each other.

The prenatal period is a time when the midwife can help the mother to prepare for the upcoming birth experience by helping her to be ready mentally, emotionally, and physically. This may be accomplished through discussions, sharing emotions, and the passing on of skills and techniques that the mother or parents may use to help them through labor. Similarly, the midwife will help the pregnant woman prepare for mothering by sharing information and skills that support breastfeeding and the health of mother and baby in the postnatal (after the birth) period.

A midwife's primary role in prenatal care is to encourage, facilitate, and nurture the mother or parents in her/their efforts to do this work. Midwives also provide thorough physical care and non-invasive prenatal assessment.

Midwives hold the belief that the most important prenatal care a woman can receive is the care she gives herself—eating well, resting adequately, avoiding environmental hazards and other factors that can affect the baby's development, and educating herself about the process through which she is going.

Preconception Care

Sometimes a midwife's care begins before a baby has been conceived. Many parents are beginning to realize the role a healthy pregnancy can play in having a healthy baby. Therefore, they want to get it right from the start. They will approach a midwife for information on ways they might prepare themselves for pregnancy. Occasionally a couple will feel more comfortable with the idea of becoming pregnant if they know they have a care provider lined up to work with them when the time arrives.

Often couples who have had difficulty conceiving or maintaining a pregnancy will contact a midwife for help in these areas. Midwives are skilled at conception counseling, often having excellent solutions for conception problems, and midwives are also able to provide suggestions for women who have miscarried before, helping them to prevent further miscarriages.

The First Trimester

Pregnancy, although one continuous process, is commonly divided into three trimesters for descriptive convenience, and perhaps as a way for women to mark the passing time. In fact, there do seem to be distinctive phases or themes that women go through during pregnancy in terms of their needs and concerns, as well as the baby's growth patterns. The first trimester, which is from conception through the thirteenth week, is the time that all of the baby's body parts—the organs, limbs, nervous system, etc.—are formed. The first trimester is the ideal time to begin working with a midwife as she can teach you ways to care for yourself that provide you and your baby with the optimal chances for wellness and healthy development. Although not all problems are preventable, many are. Maternal nutrition may be the single most important factor in preventing these conditions. First-trimester midwifery care with attention to nutrition is also excellent for preventing, or at least reducing, such common complaints as nausea (morning sickness), insomnia, anxiety, and fatigue.

Once you begin to work with a midwife, one of the first things she might have you do is to fill out a "diet diary," a record of all that you eat and drink for a specified number of days. She will look this over with you once it is completed, and help you to see what foods and nutrients your diet may be lacking.

A midwife can help to soothe first-trimester concerns, which may be particularly pronounced for first-time parents.

Your First Prenatal Appointment: Getting to Know You

At this visit it will be your midwife's primary goal to get to know you through talking with you as well as through gathering a comprehensive health history. At this meeting she will determine what areas, if any, are of specific concern or need special attention. The health history is a standard questionnaire that creates a physical picture including past and current illnesses, gynecological history (i.e., length and duration of your menstrual cycle), family medical history relevant to childbearing, and history of past pregnancies, miscarriages, and so on. From this, your midwife will also help you figure out the approximate time your baby is due.

By chronicling your health history, your midwife will gain insights into your general health patterns, and this may influence suggestions she makes for your care or areas she feels warrant further investigation. For example, a woman with a history of anemia and hypoglycemia, or a history of eating disorders, will need to learn to pay extra attention to maintaining excellent nutrition during pregnancy and after the baby is born. The beautiful thing about midwifery care is that it tends to be nourishing rather than judgmental. It is an educational approach that supports women in taking optimal care of themselves here and now, rather than in placing them into health and disease categories. Midwifery care is also preventive care, so that a woman who may have had problems in a particular area in the past might find that her midwife can provide her with advice that can prevent or reduce this problem early on. Finally, if you do have medical problems that are revealed in this heath history, and which make you ineligible for a low-risk midwifery or homebirth practice, the midwife will clearly inform you of this, and assist you in making other arrangements.

Addressing Concerns and Anxieties
At the initial prenatal visit your midwife will ask about fears or concerns you have about pregnancy, birth, and

particularly homebirth if this is your first baby or first homebirth. This visit will also include some discussion of why you are choosing to work with a midwife, and why you are choosing a homebirth. If you do have concerns about pregnancy or about the choices you are making, she can point you in the direction of excellent resources, engage you in discussions that help to calm your anxieties, or help you to find other options for care that make you feel more secure. A midwife pays attention to a mother's comfort levels throughout the pregnancy, and in part, this is what makes her an effective support person at your birth—she has learned to recognize when you are anxious, she has learned to help you find courage and comfort at these times, and she has learned to support you in ways that are most appropriate for who you are.

Your First Physical Examination

Most midwives will gather physical exam information simply by spending time with you and doing basic assessments such as listening to your lungs and heart, and checking your pulse and blood pressure. A complete physical exam can provide you and your midwife with what is referred to as "baseline" information—that is, what is "normal" for you. The initial exam will be a more comprehensive exam than you will have at subsequent prenatal visits unless otherwise warranted. The value of such baseline information will be enhanced if you begin your prenatal care early in the pregnancy.

Another component of the initial exam might be a breast exam, wherein the mother is taught to examine her own breasts (though I do not encourage this to be done throughout the pregnancy as the breasts are changing so much). Breast self-exams are considered an effective and important method in the early detection of cancer, and of course early detection means early treatment.

Most midwives, prior to any physical exam, will first try to ascertain your level of comfort at being touched. Touch is an important component of a midwife's techniques for providing comfort and support during labor, and therefore to her ability to provide care. Above all, midwives regard a right to a woman's privacy and ultimately see her as her own primary care provider. They strive to support women in making informed choices and taking responsibility for their own well-being. Midwives will often begin a physical exam by explaining exactly what they will do, what it means, and—as they do the exam—what they are finding and what that means for the individual woman and her baby. Going from your head to your feet she will notice the health of your hair and teeth, your skin, will do the previously mentioned assessments, and will also pay attention to anything unusual in your response to being touched. If you are far enough along in your pregnancy for her to feel your baby and listen to the baby's heartbeat, she will do these things and assist you in learning to do them as well.

As part of an initial physical exam, some midwives will do a vaginal exam. This is done to assess pelvic size, to make certain there are no pelvic deformities that would interfere with birth, to determine how the mother responds to personal touch from the midwife, and to make note of the appearance of the vulva, so that at birth if the mother does have any lacerations, the midwife will have a sense of how things looked before so she can help put them back together.

There is some question as to the necessity of a vaginal exam early in pregnancy because the pelvis is a movable, stretchable structure which expands late in pregnancy and during birth to accommodate the baby's head, so unless a woman has an abnormally small pelvis, early measurement is not a clear indicator of ability to birth. Perhaps the most useful reason to do a vaginal examination prenatally is to help women learn how to use their pelvic floor muscles by showing them where they are, how to contract and relax them, and by helping them to identify where they hold pelvic tension, which many women do. Many women have little knowledge about their reproductive anatomy, and this is a perfect time to learn.

Prenatal Testing
Prenatal testing refers to laboratory tests that are done either by your midwife, by a doctor, or at a lab to which you are referred. This includes blood tests to determine your blood type and Rh factor, a screen for syphilis, your red and white blood cell counts, a screen for German measles, and a test for hepatitis B and HIV. She might also request that you have vaginal cultures taken (a sample of your vaginal and cervical secretions is taken with a cotton swab) and evaluated for other sexually transmitted diseases that could affect you, your baby, or your midwife. Some of the information gained from these tests can help your midwife make recommendations that can improve your prenatal health.

Some midwives choose not to incorporate any medical testing in their practices, and some parents prefer this, relying solely on an intuitive and common sense approach to prenatal health. Such midwifery care can be effective and successful, and your combined intuitive sense of how things are going can be accurate. If you choose to follow such an approach or if you work with a midwife who does not use any prenatal screening, it is important for you to fully understand what you are not having done, and to be willing to take full personal responsibility for the outcome.

Most midwives do not incorporate testing for fetal abnormalities into their practices unless specifically requested by the parents, or if there seems to be a medical need to do so, such as a family history of certain problems, or if there has been exposure to teratogenic substances (those which can cause abnormal embryonic or fetal development) and the mother wants to know whether the baby is okay, and/or possibly wants to terminate the pregnancy if the baby is not. Your midwife will refer you to a medical practice for tests such as alpha-fetal protein (AFP), ultrasonography, amniocentesis, and chorionic villi sampling (CVS).

Regular Prenatal Visits during Your First Trimester

After your initial visit, which may be as long as two hours, you will have regular visits on a monthly basis throughout your first trimester. Each of these visits, which will range in length from about an hour to an hour and a half, will consist of time for a prenatal exam, talk, and education. Prior to the second trimester it is hard to hear the baby's heartbeat without the aid of electronic equipment, and the baby is still too small to feel by abdominal palpation. At each prenatal visit your midwife is likely to include some of the following tests which are described here:

Blood pressure—Your midwife will check your blood pressure or will have you do so if she has a self-checking blood pressure cuff. Very low blood pressure can let you know that you might need to improve your iron levels or that you need more exercise. High blood pressure can indicate stress or physiological problems that need further attention.

Pulse—An elevated pulse could indicate anxiety, the need for either relaxation or exercise, or an infection.

Urinalysis—Using a "dipstick," a chemically impregnated test strip, in a sample of your urine, you and your midwife can check kidney function by the presence of protein, whether you are getting enough carbohydrates by the presence of ketones, and sugar metabolism by the presence of glucose. At any given time a pregnant mother may have some traces of these in her urine with no problems present; but the persistent presence of any of these may be cause for further evaluation. Some midwives will use more extensive urine test strips which check for the presence of leukocytes (white blood cells) and nitrites (a byproduct of bacterial breakdown), both of which may indicate a urinary tract infection, or strips which test for other substances.

Weight—Weighing pregnant women has become a ritual in this culture, and one that I think we could easily do without. Lack of weight gain in a pregnant woman is usually readily apparent to anyone with a bit of experience in the area, and a "good" weight gain does not ensure proper nutrition. Therefore, much more emphasis ought to be placed on dietary assessment and improving nutrition. In my practice a woman can tell me her weight if she wants to, but I do not have women routinely weigh at prenatals, and I encourage women not to watch the scale at home either.

In addition to the above, your midwife will ask you questions about how you are feeling—whether you have been experiencing headaches, nausea, swelling, dizziness, blurred vision, pain, or other symptoms. If so, she will assess symptoms further and provide you with suggestions or, if needed, a referral for medical care. She will also ask you about your eating habits and appetite, as well as exercise, as midwives know that a healthy diet and adequate exercise are important for a healthy pregnancy, birth, and postpartum.

Midwives are skilled in prenatal counseling, and are familiar with the many issues women face as they welcome a baby into their lives. A midwife can provide creative suggestions for coping with stress and help you to find personal and community resources to help meet your needs. Midwives who are mothers can be especially empathetic to the emotional upheaval that a pregnancy can bring. If you have a job outside the home, or other children whose needs compete with your ability to focus on caring for yourself, your midwife will help you find ways to make the time to eat well, rest, and exercise.

Your midwife will recommend books to read about pregnancy and birth and will help you find prenatal classes (or she might teach these herself).

Miscarriage

For women with a history of miscarriage, midwifery care can be excellent preventative care. Should you begin to have mild spotting or cramping, a midwife can often provide suggestions to arrest these symptoms and provide emotional support, as she will understand that this is a frightening and sad experience to go through. If you are clearly miscarrying, she will assess the severity of your bleeding, and if it seems appropriate and safe to continue the procedure at home, she may be willing to do so. If the situation is complicated, she will suggest that you go to the hospital, and will continue to support you there. She will also provide follow-up care and suggestions for healing, both physically and emotionally.

Contacting Your Midwife

At your initial prenatal visit your midwife will provide you with numbers where she can be reached 24 hours a day, 7 days a week. Most midwives have pagers, and some also maintain an answering service. Your midwife will arrange for another midwife to take calls for her when she takes vacations or if she is attending another client when you need her.

Though your midwife will be available for you at any time in case of an emergency, there may be times when you just want to ask a few questions or chat. Your midwife will make time to talk with you, but it is important for you to be understanding and not take it personally if she says she must return your call at a later time. Midwives have to take care of themselves and their own families, too, and most midwives work from their homes, so this is likely to be where you are calling.

Medical Back-Up

In some states where midwives are licensed, midwives are required to have their clients see a physician, usually an obstetrician, for a prescribed number of prenatal visits. This doctor, or someone in the doctor's practice, will then be available to provide medical care should a problem arise prenatally or at birth. In states where midwifery is legal but not licensed, or where it is not legal, it is up to the midwife whether she will require the mother to see a physician prenatally, and up to both of you to arrange back-up care for the birth. The mother should have the final decision as to whether she wants medical involvement in her care. Some midwives and parents prefer the security of such an arrangement, knowing that should an emergency arise they have prearranged medical care (provided that their doctor is on-call) at the hospital. In some practices, you might be able to see the nurse-midwives for your prenatal visits to the obstetrician's office, and should transport to the hospital become a necessity at birth, you can see the CNMs in the hospital unless there is an emergency which requires the obstetrician.

Midwives will usually know whether there are obstetricians in the area that are receptive to midwifery/homebirth clients, and they will refer you specifically to such care providers if available.

The Second Trimester

The second trimester is the time between 14 and 28 weeks of pregnancy. During this time most midwives will see you on a monthly basis unless more appointments are necessary.

New Sensations, Excellent Support

At this stage you are probably feeling excited about your baby and are probably no longer feeling some of the first-trimester discomforts. Soon you will feel your baby's movements, and the pregnancy will become more tangible to you and to others, especially as your growing belly becomes more visible. This can be a joyous time, and also a time when you have new concerns. Frequently as your belly begins to publicly announce your pregnancy, well-meaning friends, neighbors, relatives, and even total strangers will begin to offer unsolicited advice, comments, and birth stories. And people are notorious for telling pregnant women all the horror stories they can think of! At this time your midwife can be an excellent source of support as she encourages you to form your own sense of confidence in your body. She can also dispel some of the gossip you hear. It is a good idea to let your midwife know about the things people are telling you so that she can help prevent you from forming misconceptions about the birthing process.

Physical Exam in the Second Trimester

During the second trimester your baby's body becomes increasingly easier to feel through abdominal palpations and it becomes easier to hear the heartbeat with a fetoscope. These will become regular parts of your prenatal visits in addition to the tests mentioned for first-trimester visits.

Feeling the baby—Palpation is the art of determining the baby's position in your womb with the hands. Most women love this part of the prenatal visit, when they share with the midwife where they feel the baby is, or the midwife helps the parents to learn to recognize the baby's position by feel. This is probably the most ancient part of the prenatal ritual—midwives all over the world, throughout time—feeling where the baby is with their hands, while massaging baby and mother. In my practice I use a pleasantly scented massage oil on the mom's belly and use this part of the prenatal visit as a time to help her relax and tune into her baby. This is a key time to involve fathers and other family members into the prenatal experience by helping them connect with the baby. While feeling your baby, your midwife might try to give an educated guess as to your baby's size and assess the amount of amniotic fluid present.

Fetal Heart Tones—Most midwives will listen to the baby's heart beat—known as auscultation—during each prenatal visit to ascertain the number of beats per minute and to make sure that this is within a normal range. This also gives the midwife something to compare the heart rate to during labor. Most midwives use a fetoscope to hear the heartbeat. This is a specially designed stethoscope that slightly amplifies the heart sound, and does not use electronics or sound waves as does the Doppler. With a fetoscope the heartbeat cannot usually be detected until about 18 weeks of pregnancy, so some midwives also have a Doppler so that they can hear the baby's heartbeat very early if necessary.

Fundal Height Measurement—With a tape measure your midwife will measure the distance in centimeters from the top of your pubic bone to the top of your uterus (the "fundus"). This is a measurement of uterine growth. You will likely notice this growth without any measurement, as will your midwife. However, taking this measurement provides an objective chart of your uterine growth pattern, which also usually reflects the baby's growth pattern. Generally the measurement in centimeters is approximately equal to your weeks of pregnancy; therefore at 28 weeks pregnancy your fundal measurement is likely to be between 26 and 30 centimeters. However, mothers may vary even more than this. Your midwife will primarily be looking for consistent growth as a sign of wellness.

Attention to Diet and Lifestyle

During the second trimester your midwife will continue to follow up on your diet, your exercise habits, and your concerns, helping you to understand the baby's needs and your own. She will also discuss family matters with you, such as your relationship with your mate and your children, as these relationships can impact on your wellness and preparation for birth. She will also talk with you and your partner about sex during pregnancy, and the benefit of a loving sexual relationship for a healthy birth. If you are not yet taking childbirth preparation classes, she might suggest some teachers in your area.

At this time she will further discuss prenatal testing options such as prenatal Rhogam if you are Rh-negative. Midwifery philosophy is based on the concept of informed choice, and this can only happen if you are informed. Therefore midwives will let you know what is available and the pros and cons of the different options.

Learning about Your Body and Birth

The second trimester is a ripe time to discuss birth—the physiology of the process, the personal significance of the experience, pain and fear, problems that could arise and how to prevent these, what you will do in case of a complication, and support measures for labor and birth. Your midwife will help you to learn more about your pelvic muscles, how they work during labor, and how to do pelvic floor exercises. These exercises can help you not only be well toned for birth, but also help you to be able to relax during labor in order to facilitate the birth. It is also a rich time to begin to visualize a healthy, well-nourished baby emerging from your body in a beautiful birth experience.

Involving the Family in Prenatal Care

During this time your midwife will make a concerted effort to involve family members in the pregnancy process as well as in discussions about birth and the new baby. She will help foster communication between you and the baby, and encourage the dad or other significant partner and siblings to talk to the baby as well. Numerous studies have revealed that communication with the baby in the womb is not only received by the baby, but is a wonderful way to begin to build relationships with this new person who has joined your family. Should you plan to have siblings be present at the birth, this is the time to begin to prepare them for that event, showing them videos and books, talking with them, and letting them express their concerns or ideas. Children often have misconceptions about birth, and merely dispelling these with accurate information can help them feel comfortable about attending.

Comfort Measures

As you come to the end of your second trimester, you may begin to experience some digestive difficulties or other complaints. Many late pregnancy problems can be prevented or minimized with the excellent prenatal care that you give yourself. Your midwife will usually be able to provide you with suggestions and information to reduce discomforts that do arise. If any serious complications arise during the second trimester, your midwife will help you find appropriate medical referrals, and in the case of emergencies, she will support you as you seek medical care.

While your midwife will spend a lot of time with you, she can't tell you everything there is to know, nor can she prepare your body, mind, and heart for the experience. It is therefore up to you to read, research, attend classes, and do the personal preparation that is so essential to a healthy experience.

The Third Trimester

The third trimester extends from the 29th week of pregnancy until the birth. During this time your prenatal visits will become increasingly more frequent. From the 28th through the 32nd week your visits will continue to be monthly; from the 32nd through 36th weeks your visits will be every two weeks, and after that your visits will be weekly until the baby is born. If you go much past your expected due time, your midwife will probably want to see you more often.

The Home Visit

If you are planning to birth at home, your midwife and her assistant(s) will come to your home about three or four weeks before you are due for a "home visit." They might request that everyone you plan to have at the birth be there for this visit. One of the primary reasons for the home visit is that your birth attendants know how to find your home—a particularly important factor if you call them to your birth in the middle of the night! Also important is that a home visit connects your home with the care you receive from your midwife which, until now, has been at her home or office. Prior to the visit, probably early in your third trimester, she will give you a list of supplies with instructions on where to find them. The home visit allows the midwives to see if your home is ready for a baby, if your supplies are in order, and if the area for birthing is clean and well organized. If you are uncertain where in your home you might like to birth, your midwives can help make suggestions about areas that seem comfortable.

Support during Late Pregnancy

Nutrition late in pregnancy is as important as ever—what you consume impacts the growth and development of the baby's brain and the baby's stores of iron. You are preparing your body to be well nourished for the demanding physical work of labor. Frequently, however, women are bored with food after so many months of eating "extra well," and your body might not be digesting large meals as easily. At this time your midwife can be a great source of inspiration and ideas for foods that are wholesome, nutritious, light, and easy to prepare. She can help you find recipes and make suggestions for improving digestion

Similarly, exercise in late pregnancy can become more difficult, particularly if you are not generally accustomed to exercise. She will try to help you find ways of maintaining physical activity so that you can enjoy your body and be well prepared for birth.

The Prenatal Exam during the Third Trimester
During late pregnancy the prenatal exam routine will be the same as during the second trimester, but your midwife may pay extra attention to blood pressure changes, swelling, and any signs or symptoms that might herald a problem. Though these are relatively rare, early detection of problems can lead to preventative and remedial measures before a problem becomes serious. If you've already had prenatal blood tests and vaginal cultures done, most midwives will not request any further testing. Some midwives will request a test for Beta-Strep, a vaginal infection that can be present and cause problems for the baby, but this is not routinely done by all midwives (nor by all obstetricians or nurse-midwives). If you have had this infection, or if you have herpes, testing might be done to determine whether infection is present around the time of birth. If it is, you can make plans for where you feel the safest place will be for your baby to be born. Your midwife will also pay more attention to the position your baby is in. If you are planning a homebirth and are unable to have a midwife at home if the baby is

breech, you will want to begin to make other arrangements well before you are due. Your midwife will recommend safe and natural methods for helping the baby to turn, and will help you to make other arrangements should a homebirth not remain an option.

Some midwives like to do an internal exam late in pregnancy, particularly if they've not done one with the mother before. This is done to assess the mother's comfort with her body, her ability to relax her pelvic and vaginal muscles, and her ability to be uninhibited in front of the midwives. They also feel whether the head is engaged or the cervix is beginning to become soft or to dilate. Unless the midwife is uncertain about the baby's position (i.e., whether there is a head or bottom in the pelvis)—or another specific question—this is not a necessary exam, and the choice of whether she wants it done should be up to the mother. Some women like to know that their body is beginning to soften and dilate in preparation for birth; other women would rather just wait and see, or would prefer to avoid an internal exam unless it's needed.

Childbirth Education

If by your third trimester you have not taken childbirth education classes, some midwives will now insist that you do so. In addition, your midwife will spend much of your visits together talking with you about labor, birth, and the care of yourself and your baby after the birth. She will make sure that you know when to call her and how to reach her. She will encourage you to arrange for supervision for the other children that you plan to have at the birth, as well as to have help lined up for yourself after the birth. She will also help prepare you for breastfeeding and some of the emotional changes you might expect in the postpartum period.

If you are planning a homebirth, your midwife will teach you about what to do in case your baby is coming fast and your midwife has not yet arrived.

Your midwife will also want to make certain that you have a thorough plan in case of emergency, including knowing relevant emergency numbers and the route to the nearest hospital or emergency center that has the capability of dealing with obstetric and neonatal complications. If she is familiar with the area in which you live, she will likely be familiar with the hospitals, but if not, she can help you come up with a list of questions for emergency back-up facilities so that you can do the research yourself. As babies can come earlier than expected, she will likely want you to have such a plan established by the time of your home visit. At this time she might suggest that if you want a pediatrician to see your baby after the birth, you should find one. Midwives can often make referrals for pediatricians that are supportive of homebirth and open-minded to alternative medical care, if this is your preference.

Realistic Expectations for Birth

Because birth cannot be planned, and problems do occasionally arise that require medical care, your midwife will help you to clarify your expectations so that they are realistic and not rigid. This is important whether you are planning to give birth at home or in a hospital. Having realistic expectations will help you to maintain the flexibility that is so literally necessary for giving birth.

DURING LABOR AND BIRTH

The long-awaited time has finally come and you will soon be welcoming your baby into your arms. This section is primarily geared toward women having their babies at home with direct-entry midwives.

Labor

During late pregnancy your midwife will advise you to call her when you think your labor has begun. She will teach you the signs of labor. She will also teach you about ways to cope with the excitement and anxiety of early labor. Staying relaxed from the onset will also help as your labor becomes very active.

Early Labor

When you call your midwife at your time of labor, she will chat with you on the phone for some time, listening to the tones in your voice, and—if you are having contractions— listening to how long they last and how you are responding to them. She will ask you about the signs of labor that you are having, and she will want to know if the baby is moving well, and how you are feeling. From this conversation she will usually be able to deduce about how far along you are in labor and whether it is time for her to come and be with you. While midwives will generally encourage parents to get through early labor themselves, your midwife will come if you feel you need help handling labor. Also, a midwife would rather come early than miss your birth.

If she knows that you are in early labor, she will encourage you to get some rest if at all possible, particularly if it is late evening or during the night. Sometimes first time parents get so excited when they think labor has begun that they will not rest and relax even if it is 2 A.M. A wise midwife will know that this can leave a woman very tired if she happens to continue to labor throughout the next day or longer, and therefore will try to get you to conserve your energy. If you seem anxious, your midwife might even suggest a massage or a glass of wine to help you relax.

Of course, if your labor seems in full force and you are handling the sensations of labor comfortably, then she will just encourage you to keep on with whatever you are doing, and to go about your daily business. If you enter labor with your bag of waters breaking, then your midwife will ascertain from you whether the fluids were clear (rather than stained with meconium) and she will provide you with general recommendations for hygiene, particularly if you are not already having contractions.

Throughout the time you are in early labor, which can be as short as an hour (or less) or as long as 24 hours (or more), your midwife will remain in close touch with you. As long as you seem to be healthy, taking care of yourself, and coping well with labor, she will merely stay in touch with you by phone to check in with how you're doing. If she lives close by or is in your neighborhood, she might even stop by.

Active Labor

Once your labor becomes active and contractions are close together, your midwife will come to be with you. When she arrives, either alone or with assistant(s), she will quietly assume her role as support for you. She will visually assess the environment to make sure that it appears both nourishing for you and ready for the birth, and she will attend to you in whatever ways you need at the moment—usually with just some comfort measures and reassurances—or perhaps just a calm presence. As the labor becomes very strong, male partners are usually quite relieved and reassured by the arrival of the midwife, but a sensitive midwife will be sure not to usurp the intimate role of the father, and will encourage him to continue to provide support. If needed, your midwife may show both of you some techniques and positions that are effective for working with the birth process, and she will encourage you to find the resources you have within yourself as a birthing woman.

The Midwife's Supplies

In addition to the supplies you have gathered, your midwife will bring her own supplies and equipment to your birth. Most midwives carry many more items than they ever use, specifically emergency supplies, but they are helpful to have on hand when needed.

The following is a typical list of supplies that a midwife might carry:

- fetoscope
- watch
- blood pressure cuff
- stethoscope
- sterile gloves
- sterile gauze pads
- scissors
- hemostats
- umbilical cord clamps
- bulb syringe
- DeLee suction device
- heating pad
- infant scale and tape measure
- medications (and syringes, alcohol swabs, etc.) and/or botanical preparations for treating hemorrhages
- urine testing strips

- oxygen unit and infant resuscitation equipment
- suturing equipment
- herbs for other purposes

Keeping an Eye on Vital Signs

When your midwife arrives, you can expect her to check your vital signs as well as listen to the baby's heartbeat. She will ask you if you've been drinking enough fluids and will make sure that you are urinating regularly so that a full bladder doesn't impede your labor. Some midwives will routinely check blood pressure and pulse periodically throughout labor, others will do so only if you have had previous problems with blood pressure, or if infection or another problem is suspected. Nearly all midwives will check fetal heart tones throughout labor, checking more frequently as labor progresses.

Some midwives will check your dilation upon arrival at your house, and then will check it periodically. Others will check only if it seems necessary or if you request that she see how far dilated you are. Most midwives, even those still in training, can tell about how far a labor has progressed just by observing the mother and listening to the sounds she is making. This ability to assess labor without a vaginal examination was put to the test in England when individual midwives were shown films of laboring women at different stages. The midwives were consistently accurate in their assessments. A midwife also knows that dilation doesn't necessarily follow a steady curve—that a woman can go very quickly from three centimeters to completely dilated, or slowly from eight centimeters to completely dilated. Stage of dilation is of secondary importance to how the mother and baby are doing with the labor, unless labor progress seems to have stopped for an inordinately long period of time, or if it is going extremely slowly.

All of the midwife's findings during labor will be carefully recorded on a labor record.

Labor Support and Long Labors

Depending upon how much labor support you need, your midwife will either find an unobtrusive spot where she can be available to you if you need her, or she will be right there helping you through contractions with helpful ideas, comfort measures, reassurance, and encouragement. During a long labor your midwife will also continue to make sure that you are eating well in order to maintain energy, and that you are drinking fluids and resting. She may suggest things to take your mind off of labor for awhile, such as a funny movie, or she may encourage you to sip some wine or use other natural techniques to promote rest. Sometimes, just taking the edge off for awhile can really leave you refreshed and renewed. These simple measures alone can often allow a woman to safely labor for a long period of time without compromise.

Birth

When the labor has become advanced and birth is close at hand, your midwife or her assistant will set up their supplies. If you are birthing at home, they will put their supplies somewhere easily movable so that you can birth in the spot or room most comfortable to you.

Woman-Centered Birthing

Though your midwife is there to help guide you safely through the birth process, the midwife herself will be taking most of her clues from you, working to help you give birth the way that you want, and supporting you to be as comfortable and actively engaged as possible. This is the heart of woman-centered birthing. While you may look to her for guidance, she will also look to you so that she may guide you appropriately, and she will help you to follow your own instincts. If she perceives that something is not working to your advantage—such as your position—she will facilitate what it is that you are trying to do. But her ultimate goal, aside from having a healthy mother and a healthy baby, is that you feel empowered by birthing, and that you be able to labor and birth as a unique expression of yourself.

Family Involvement at the Birth
During birth your midwife will make an effort to involve your family in the process. It can be helpful for each of the other children to have something special to do at the birth. such as noticing what time the baby is born, giving mom sips of drinks, bringing mom a cool cloth, or being the one to announce whether the baby is a boy or a girl.

Pushing Your Baby into the World
During the phase of labor when you are actually pushing your baby into the world, your midwife will be listening to the baby's heartbeat slightly more frequently, she will be offering you sips of fluids, and she will be helping you to work with your body. Your midwife will explain to you the positions and techniques that encourage the baby to come down your birth canal and be born.

Preventing Vaginal Tears
At this point your midwife will either sit very close to you (often near your legs), simply observing your vaginal opening

as the baby is being born, or she will apply warm compresses or gently massage oil on your perineum, to facilitate the stretching of the vaginal opening and to prevent the tearing of the perineum.

While most women—given the time to stretch slowly as the baby emerges—will not tear, some midwives feel that intervention at this point is beneficial. This depends upon the beliefs of the midwife, and on your personal preference—some birthing women like both compresses and perineal massage, some don't want to be touched at that time. It is your birth and you get to decide.

Welcome, Baby

Your midwife will have warmed towels on hand, with which you can dry the baby immediately after she/he is born. Her other equipment will be nearby in the rare case of problem, but it is her attention that will be most present. What actually transpires at the moment of birth is based on your level of active involvement and your desires, as well as the philosophy of the midwife attending you. It is optimal to have discussed your wishes with her well before labor begins, and to remind her of any special plans at the onset of labor. Although birth cannot be planned, if she has an idea about your preferences, she can do her best to provide the individual touches you want.

Generally the room will be made warm before the actual birth so that skin-to-skin contact between parents and baby is possible, and most midwives will also dim lights so that the baby is not made uncomfortable by the transition from the dim womb to a bright room. Some midwives will also have a newborn cap on hand to place on the baby's head to maintain the baby's temperature.

As the baby comes out, your midwife will either encourage you to put your hands on the baby and help her/him out yourself, or have your mate help. If you do not wish to do this, the midwife will lift the baby onto your chest or belly and cover the child lightly with a towel to keep the baby warm.

When the baby is born the midwife will not announce the sex of your baby, but will wait until you discover that for yourself, or she will encourage a sibling to take a peek and make the announcement. There will not be a rush to cut the umbilical cord, in fact many midwives prefer to wait until the placenta is out for the cord to be cut. Birth with a midwife is usually a gentle and peaceful event.

Problems at Birth

If there are problems at this time, things may be slightly different than just described. If, for example, there have been worrisome decreases in the baby's heart rate close to birth, the midwife may encourage you to push the baby out quickly once you are completely dilated. If there has been meconium present in the amniotic fluid (other than with a breech birth), the midwife will suction the baby's mouth and nose with a thin sterile tube once the head is out, but before the body has even come out. If the baby isn't breathing well, or if the heartbeat is weak, she may provide gentle stimulation by rubbing the baby's feet and back and encouraging you to do the same. If more severe problems require resuscitation efforts, she will engage in this. However, unlike what occurs in a hospital environment, any procedures will be done only because completely necessary (rather than just routinely), and the baby will never be removed from your presence. Rather, the midwife will elicit your involvement as much as possible, as midwives know that a parents' efforts of speaking to, and touching their baby can greatly improve the situation and the baby's responsiveness.

The Placenta Comes Out, Too

The placenta will usually be born within an hour of the birth, and most often within 30 minutes. While you are waiting you will simply be cuddling your baby and, perhaps, holding your baby to your breast for the first nursing, which will help to expel the placenta and control bleeding. During this time, your midwife will be keeping an eye on the baby and on you. She will offer you something to drink and eat, and will help you get comfortable holding and nursing your little one.

Once you are ready to expel the placenta she will help you do so—catching it in a bowl and setting it aside to examine later—and then she will help you to get comfortable in your bed and will tidy the area around you. At this time she will leave you alone for awhile with your immediate family to enjoy your baby and your accomplishment, while she washes her hands, fills out charts, or takes a break in the next room. She will check in periodically to make sure that all is well.

Just After the Birth

After about another 30 minutes she'll help you to get cleaned up in a shower or will rinse you off. She will have you get up to relieve yourself, and will make sure that you have something to eat and drink. She will show the placenta to you if you want to look at it, and will explain its different parts. She will then do a thorough examination of the baby, and at this time will weigh and measure him/her, while the baby is right next to you. She will give you help with breastfeeding, showing you how to get the baby to latch on if s/he hasn't already done so, and show you comfortable positions in which to nurse.

If all is well, she will answer questions, provide you with clear instructions for the first 24 hours, and leave your home. Most midwives will stay with you for a minimum of two hours after a healthy birth, longer if there have been any problems.

Care After the Birth

Midwives will make a varying number of visits back to their client's homes, depending upon the volume of clients in their practices, distance to your home, and your need for postpartum support. Postpartum care can range from visiting you once during the first week and checking in with you daily by phone, to seeing you once or more at your home during the first week (usually on the first and/or third days) and then at subsequent visits back at her office (usually two and six weeks after the birth).

In the immediate postpartum—the first few days—your midwife will give you instructions on danger signs for both you and the baby, and will make sure that you have someone to be with you for at least the first days after the birth. She will also make sure that nursing is going well, that you are healing, and she will give you instructions on basic things such as care of the umbilical cord stump.

Postpartum care during the first week can be a simple check-up on how things are going—nursing, your bleeding, how your bottom feels if there were tears, etc., or it can be an elaborate ritual of new-mother nourishment with herbal sitz baths, massage, and other complementary health practices.

If you want more elaborate postpartum care and your midwife does not include this in her services, she can still educate you about techniques you can use to make the weeks after the birth a time of special nourishment for yourself and your baby.

Some midwives who provide a six-week postpartum check will review family planning (birth control) and offer to do a pap-smear if the mother wants one done.

In all cases, your midwife will remain available to you 24 hours a day, 7 days a week for emergencies, and for answering the questions that new parents so often have. She will also continue to do so for at least the first six weeks after the birth. Regardless of how many visits she provides, all midwives recognize that the transition to parenting does not end at birth but merely begins there. Midwives are frequently in touch with their clients and often are still answering breastfeeding and parenting questions well into the first year after the birth.

Breastfeeding

Midwife clients have excellent success with breastfeeding, with most being able to nurse their baby within the first hours after birth, and to continue long-term nursing. Sometimes they are able to breastfeed even as long as the international breastfeeding average of over two years. This is the case for both stay-at-home mothers and those who work outside the home who wish to breastfeed. Midwives are able to help women work through many breastfeeding problems, and if a problem is beyond their scope, they will enlist the help of La Leche League leaders or lactation consultants.

Complications and Emergencies

Most births go smoothly, and small problems that come

up are often resolvable at home if attended to promptly. Unexpected catastrophic emergencies are exceptionally rare during childbirth, but a midwife does study complications extensively as part of her midwifery training, and learns how to prevent, recognize, and respond to emergencies. Midwives are capable of administering treatment for many emergency situations, and of working to keep the mother and baby in stable condition until medical help is obtained, should this be necessary. However, even with the most advanced technologies, not all problems can be anticipated. When you plan a homebirth and work with a midwife, this is a responsibility you must assume.

Prior to birth, your midwife should discuss with you what to expect in case of an emergency and let you know what procedures she will follow. Together, you will come up with a plan, based on where you live, as to how and where to get medical help quickly.

Transport to the Hospital

If your midwife thinks transport to the hospital is necessary, she will discuss the matter thoroughly. Your midwife will make every possible effort to help you achieve the birth you want within parameters that are safe for you and your baby. In the case of an emergency, your midwife will discuss options with you as she takes necessary action, such as calling emergency services or performing neonatal resuscitation.

If you must transport, your midwife will likely go to the hospital with you. If she is practicing in a state where the medical and legal establishments are hostile to midwives, she might go in as a labor support person rather than calling herself your midwife. However, midwives generally choose to be direct about their role in order to provide thorough background information to the hospital staff, and to make a statement for the quality of care that midwives provide. These issues will need to be discussed far in advance so you know what to expect and know whether your midwife will need to be protected from legal harassment.

In a state where midwifery is legal, your midwife will be able to be open about her professional involvement. While direct-entry midwives cannot usually provide hands-on care in the hospital, they can continue to provide emotional and physical support, as well as act as an advocate for you, explaining procedures and options.

If you have a back-up doctor, your mate or midwife will have phoned in advance, stating that you are going to the hospital, and she/he will hopefully meet you there.

The Pediatrician

Some midwives require their clients to take the baby to a pediatrician within the first week after birth, while others will leave this matter to the parents' discretion. If there seems to be a medical problem that warrants the attention of a pediatrician, then your midwife will certainly recommend that you take the baby to be seen. Your midwife will also let you know the appropriate time frame for obtaining newborn tests such as the PKU test (tests for phenylketonuria, thyroid disease, and sometimes other conditions) and any other tests that might be indicated. Most midwives do not provide newborn testing at home beyond the initial thorough newborn exam, and brief checks at the postpartum visits—though some do provide PKU testing as part of routine postpartum care.

MIDWIFE-RUN CLINICS AND BIRTHING CENTERS

In some states, direct-entry midwives can direct and staff clinics and birthing centers, just as can CNMs and MDs. If you are having your baby with a midwife in a birthing center, the care will be very similar to that just described. The main difference is that you will go to the clinic or center for your prenatal care and you will not have a home visit at your house prior to the birth. Your midwife will meet you at the center when you are in labor, rather than at your home, and postpartum follow-up will generally be back at the center.

It is important that you clearly understand the limits and regulations pertaining to the place you choose to birth, as well as the limits placed on your attendants, well before the time of birth so that you can have a clear sense of how different situations might be handled. See Chapter 5 "Choosing A Midwife," for ideas on interviewing midwives.

BEYOND PREGNANCY AND BIRTH

Midwives are able to provide a broad range of what is generally referred to as "well-woman" gynecological care. That is, women's health care that is based on prevention, education, and general physical assessment rather than emergency gynecological care and surgery. Midwives provide sex education to adolescents and teenagers, provide family planning counseling, do breast exams, teach women to do breast self-exams, and perform routine gynecological testing such as pap-smears. Some midwives fit birth control devices such as cervical caps, and all are a rich source of information and support to women as they go through the various stages of reproductive development, from the onset of puberty through menopause.

Choosing the Care You Want

You've read this far and now perhaps you're interested in working with a midwife—maybe even having a homebirth—but you still have questions. What exactly can the midwife do? What if you hemorrhage? What about pain relief in labor? What if you need a cesarean section? This chapter will provide you with answers to some of these questions.

WHAT ARE YOU LOOKING FOR?

Having a baby can be a joyous, nurturing, and empowering experience. Most women have come to expect childbearing to be a medicalized experience from start to finish. But is this what you really want? It is most important that you make the choice that is right for *you*. Look over this list of questions to ask yourself.

- What type of medical care do I generally seek when I am ill (Western, holistic, self-administered)?
- Do I feel that childbirth is a normal, healthy, and safe process, or a (dangerous) medical event?
- If I had my baby at home and something happened to the baby, how might I feel about my choice?
- If I had my baby in the hospital and something happened to the baby, how might I feel?
- Who do I want with me at prenatal visits? during labor and birth?
- Where would I feel most secure laboring? birthing?
- Do I want to be able to move around freely during labor?
- Do I want to be able to eat and drink freely during labor?

- How do I feel about medical interventions such as external/internal electronic fetal monitoring, regular vaginal examinations, IVs, pitocin, amniotomy, forceps, episiotomy?
- Am I willing to try laboring without pain medication?
- Do I want to hold my baby immediately after birth?
- How do I feel about breastfeeding my baby?
- Do I want to be home during or right after the birth?
- What other things are important to me?

Further into your pregnancy your answers and beliefs might change, but in order to choose the type of care provider that is appropriate for you to get started with, you must have a general sense of your own beliefs and the direction in which you want to go. If you choose a care setting or care provider that doesn't work for you, you can make a change even late in the pregnancy, and you can always go to the hospital during labor if you decide homebirth isn't what you want.

Can You Work with a Direct-Entry Midwife?

Any pregnant woman can work with a midwife, but in certain cases when a woman has a higher risk for complications, a DEM cannot provide primary care or offer homebirth services. She may be able to serve as a consultant for you in areas of nutrition, use complementary health methods to reduce your risk factors, or provide education and support. Some midwives are even willing to serve as a labor support person for women who need to have their babies in the hospital.

The following is a list of high-risk factors for which your midwife will screen. Those with an asterisk next to them mean that not all midwives consider this to be a risk factor, but that the situation must be evaluated individually.

- poor nutrition, poor health
- diabetes

- hypertension (high blood pressure)
- heart disease
- kidney disease
- active genital herpes at the time of birth
- previous cesarean section*
- previous stillbirth*
- history of severe hemorrhage with unknown or repeatable causes
- anemia*
- fetal distress
- infection
- toxemia
- Rh-negative mom with antibody sensitization
- polyhydramnios
- placenta previa
- breech presentation*
- multiple pregnancy*
- premature rupture of the membranes*
- premature labor (more than 3 weeks before due date)*
- postmature labor (more than 2 weeks after due date)*
- smoking*
- fifth or subsequent baby*

*Age under 16 or over 35 for first baby, or over 40 for any pregnancy

List from *Special Delivery: The Complete Guide to Informed Birth*, by Rahima Baldwin, 1979.

Birth Setting

When choosing care providers you are usually choosing your place of birth as well. In 1996, 78 percent of all home-births in the United States were attended by direct-entry midwives (the other 22 percent of births were attended by MDs, CNMs, or were attended only by the parents). Only

3 percent of CNMs (or about 200 nurse-midwives) attend homebirths in the United States. Relatively few DEMs have birthing center practices, but this number is expected to grow as midwives gain legislation to support this option.

As discussed in Chapter 1 "Midwifery and Safety," planned homebirth with a midwife has an excellent track record for safety, frequently better than that of obstetricians and hospitals, especially for low-risk women. The advantage of birthing in the hospital is having immediate access to emergency medical care should this be necessary.

The place where you birth will, to a large extent, determine the type of care you receive and the extent to which you can make choices about your care and the baby's care. Most institutions provide institutionalized care.

Midwives practice within the midwifery model of care which is inherently a "with woman" model. The needs of the mother and baby are the primary determinants of the care that is provided, and the mother—as an autonomous adult—has the right to choose the care that best suits her. Proponents of the midwifery model of care assert that the mother will have the best interest of her baby in mind, and will choose her care accordingly. In fact, it is because women are so determined to care for their babies that they have been misled into accepting medical interventions which they are told are in the best interest of their babies, but which are actually not beneficial and may even be harmful.

Midwifery Model of Care and Medical Model of Care

The midwifery and medical models of care are dramatically different approaches that direct and define what care child-bearing women receive. While there are currently steps being taken jointly by midwives, medical practitioners, and other supporters to incorporate the midwifery model of care into clinics, hospitals, and doctor's offices, midwives are still the most qualified practitioners to provide this care.

Midwifery and Medical Models of Care

Midwifery Model	Medical Model
• The woman maintains power and authority over herself.	• Power and authority are handed over to the institution.
• Responsibility is in the hands of the woman herself, shared with her midwife.	• Responsibility is assumed by the physician.
• The goal is to assist the woman toward self-care as a healthy person in a state of normalcy.	• The woman is encouraged to be dependent and is treated as potentially ill and in an abnormal state.
• The mother and baby are a unit whose medical and emotional needs are complementary; what meets needs of one meets the needs of both.	• The mother and baby are separate patients whose medical and emotional needs may conflict; the mother's emotional needs may jeopardize the baby's health.
•The woman's body is a well-functioning home for herself and her baby, with needs and workings best known by the woman herself.	• The woman's body is a mechanical organism that needs fixing, with needs and workings best known by the physician.

• Childbirth is seen as an activity that the healthy woman engages in.	• Childbirth is seen as an occasion for the provision of medical services.
• The midwife guides and educates the woman during her experience.	• The physician manages the care of the woman.
• The best prenatal care is empathetic, caring.	• The best prenatal care is objective, scientific.
• The health of the baby is ensured through the physical and emotional health of the mother her and attunement to the baby.	• The health of the baby during pregnancy is ensured through drugs, tests, and procedures.
• Labor can be short or can take several days.	• Birth must happen within 26 hours.
•Labor follows its own rhythms.	• Once labor begins it must progress steadily or intervention is necessary.
• Environmental ambience is key to safe birth.	• Environmental ambience is irrelevant.
• Labor pain is acceptable, normal.	• Labor pain is unacceptable, abnormal.
• A woman in labor can do what she feels like—moving, eating, sexual intimacy with partner, and sleeping are all appropriate.	• Confinement to bed, hooked up to machines with frequent exams by staff, is appropriate for a woman in labor.

• The midwife supports, assists.	• The doctor controls.
• The mother births the baby.	• The doctor delivers the baby.

The author wishes to credit the work of Barbara Katz Rothman in her book *In Labor: Women and Power in the Birthplace* (1982), and Robbie Davis-Floyd in her book *Birth as an American Right of Passage* (1992). In her book Davis-Floyd uses the terms "Technocratic Model of Birth" and "Holistic Model of Birth" as points of comparison. Also, thanks to Elizabeth Hallett and Karen Ehrlich, authors of the booklet *Midwife Means "With Woman"* for the format for this chart, and for their adaptation of this information.

CHOOSING THE EXPERIENCE YOU WANT

In our culture we tend to assume that the medical way is the best way because it is based on scientific truth. Yet few of us realize that not all medical decisions are in fact based on scientific evidence. A World Health Organization survey of routine obstetric interventions found that only 10 percent were justified by scientific evidence.

The following are a few of the many areas in which the medical model and midwifery model diverge in care and treatment. Frequently the approach of the medical model is based on considerations such as malpractice insurance, hospital protocol, and convenience, whereas the midwifery approach is based on the needs of individual childbearing women.

Nourishment during Labor

It is common medical practice to withhold food and drink from women in labor for fear that should an emergency cesarean be necessary, the woman will run an increased risk of aspirating vomitus while under anaesthesia. While this is a possibility, it is rare for a woman to need an emergency cesarean under general anesthesia. Conventional obstetrical practice is to allow only ice-chips for the duration of labor; intravenous fluids are considered to be sufficient nourishment should labor be long or the woman dehydrated.

Nurse-midwives may be more flexible in birthing centers allowing women to drink juice and to eat lightly in early labor.

Midwives and nurse-midwives with home-based practices and progressive birthing center practices know—both from reviewing medical literature and from clinical experience—that women who are well-nourished during labor tend to have more effective labors, are better able to cope with long labors, have a higher pain tolerance, and generally feel more energetic during and after the birth. Midwives therefore encourage their clients to eat freely of nutritious foods during labor and to drink plentifully to replace fluids and prevent dehydration.

Positions for Labor and Birth

Until recently women giving birth in hospitals have been restricted to their beds, encumbered by IV lines in their arms and fetal monitors strapped to their bellies. Thanks to the efforts of midwives, many hospitals have realized that such restriction is not only unnecessary, but is not beneficial for the mother or baby. While many hospitals still require that laboring mothers have an IV inserted, women are allowed to move around with the IV cart, which they must push along as they walk. If the baby's heart tones seem fine after a period of initial monitoring, the women may move around without the monitor, provided they wear it for at least 15 minutes each hour.

Midwives have long recognized the benefits for the mother and baby of encouraging the mother to move around freely, and for her to choose the positions that are most comfortable for her. This facilitates labor and gives the mother a sense of empowerment, reducing the need for pain relief. It can also prevent fetal distress which is associated with having laboring women lay on their backs for long periods of time.

The freedom to birth in a variety of positions further encourages birth to occur spontaneously, preventing problems such as "failure to progress," cephalopelvic disproportion (CPD), and shoulder dystocia. With midwives, labor and birthing positions include, but are not limited to, squatting, semi-sitting, kneeling, standing, side-lying, sitting on a chair or birthing stool, and reclining.

The ability to assume a variety of comfortable positions is most enhanced when women give birth at home, where they have the freedom to use all of their familiar surroundings. In this area both hospitals and birthing centers provide limited choices.

Pain/Pain Relief

Obstetrics views pain primarily as a side-effect of having a baby, which can easily be eliminated with the use of pain medications. At one hospital I was recently told that 95 percent of the women that give birth there have epidurals. I have repeatedly seen pain medication pushed on women in labor, particularly at the height of a strong contraction. Unfortunately, the risks of pain medication, while briefly explained to laboring women, are mostly glossed over. The medication is made to seem a glorious advantage over the archaic choice of feeling one's labor.

Nurse-midwives tend to view pain as a natural part of labor, and usually support and encourage women to avoid pain medication unless absolutely necessary. However, for nurse-midwives practicing in medical settings, medication is always readily available and this *can* allow for its unnecessary use.

Direct-entry midwives see pain as a natural but not inevitable aspect of birth, and encourage women to discover their abilities to cope with the sensations of labor. Midwives honor a woman's choice to receive pain medication, but they realize that these drugs are not without risks to the mother and baby. Risks include delayed labor progress, inability to effectively push the baby out, respiratory depression for the newborn, and seizures and death for the mother. Epidural anesthesia is associated with long-term back discomfort, and the drug *Fentanil* is associated with respiratory depression of the newborn, so the neonatal intensive care unit (NICU) team must be present in the room at the time of birth should the baby require intensive resuscitation efforts.

Because midwives do not carry pain medication, they cannot offer this to you, but they can offer you support, encouragement, and a host of comfort measures that usually provide immense help. Should you decide that you do want medication, or should this be necessary in a difficult labor, you can transport to the hospital where pain medication is available.

Common Interventions

In addition to IVs and external fetal monitors, a host of interventions often accompany a hospital birth with an obstetrician. Labor may actually be considered normal—even natural—though there may be interventions including amniotomy (artificial rupture of membranes), pitocin induction or augmentation, epidural, and episiotomy.

Because of their training and affiliation with doctors, hospitals, and hospital birthing centers, nurse-midwives walk in the middle of the road when it comes to interventions. Though most nurse-midwives will try to be as flexible as possible in stretching time limits and other situations for the best interest of the mother and baby, they can stretch the rules only so far. A nurse-midwife's ability to be autonomous is dependent upon where she works and with whom she practices.

Direct-entry midwives are well aware of the parameters of a healthy birth, and are fully knowledgeable regarding standard medical protocols. However, because they are devoted to serving the mother and child, not a medical institution, insurance company, or a time limit for their own convenience, midwives are able to apply such knowledge to individual situations. Furthermore, midwives know that birth proceeds best when there are no interventions. Any interventions that become necessary are done sparingly to avoid the domino effect so commonly seen in hospitals, where one intervention leads to the next.

Labor Support

Meta-analysis of ten randomized trials has shown that simply having a personal birth attendant supporting women throughout labor "is effective in reducing analgesia requirements, lowers the incidence of cesarean section and operative delivery, and improves fetal outcome" (Thornton and Lilford 1994, Wagner 1995).

Women who choose to have an obstetrician attend them in the hospital can be fairly certain that their doctor will not be available to provide labor support and that s/he will only be available for the birth itself. Your support during labor and birth will come only from any attendants you brought with you (i.e., mate, friend, professional labor support person) and occasionally from nurses.

A nurse-midwife will provide you with support and guidance during labor for as much time as she is able. This will depend on how well staffed the hospital or birthing center is when you are in labor. If she is the only midwife available for several women then you will not receive as much support as if she were caring for you at home, in which case her care might be continuous, as it is with direct-entry midwives.

Direct-entry midwives are available to women during labor, though they do encourage women to have their mate or a close friend also available for labor support. Your midwife will provide you with continuous support once she is called to attend you, encouraging and assisting you without taking over. Furthermore, midwives encourage the support and participation of your family and friends, who might be excluded in a medical setting.

Fetal Monitoring

Numerous studies have revealed that monitoring the baby's heartbeat with a fetoscope during pregnancy and labor is as effective as monitoring with electronic fetal monitors. Women may be more likely to undergo unnecessary worry and interventions, including cesarean sections, as a result of electronic fetal monitoring. When monitoring with a fetoscope is done correctly, it is a highly effective means of determining ominous variations in the heart tones. Also, there is little room for the mechanical problems associated with the machines, or complications associated with the woman being immobile as is required with both external and internal fetal monitoring.

Doctors and nurse-midwives almost universally monitor fetal heart tones with electronic external or internal fetal monitors; midwives almost universally monitor using fetoscopes.

Episiotomy

Episiotomy is the surgical incision of the perineum, the area between the vaginal opening and the anus, done to widen the vagina as the baby is being born. The incision is then stitched after the birth. The rationale behind the procedure, which is now routine in most hospitals, is to allow the baby to be born more quickly and prevent tears, as well as to prevent the vaginal muscles from becoming overstretched (preventing future vaginal and pelvic laxity). This is done in spite of increased risk of bleeding, infection, and postpartum discomfort for the mother which may last more than a year after birth and which may interfere with comfortable sex during that time.

Midwives from all backgrounds know that a woman's body is meant to stretch in order to birth her baby, and that vaginal tissue heals remarkably well. Episiotomy rates among midwives (CNMs and DEMs alike) are low, with episiotomy only being done when medically necessary. Most midwives are skilled in the repair of tears and episiotomies, but midwives can also claim that most of their clients do not tear when giving birth naturally, nor are they subject to pelvic laxity any more than women receiving episiotomies.

Bonding and Breastfeeding

Babies born in the hospital are subject to numerous routine examinations and interventions. Should even a minor problem be perceived, the baby will be separated from the mother until the medical staff feels the problem is resolved. Time for bonding is allowed if the baby seems perfectly healthy, but it is not a priority of the medical staff. Similarly, breastfeeding support varies from hospital to hospital, and while it may be superficially supported, you are also likely to be offered samples of formula and other bottle-feeding paraphernalia. There may or may not be someone on staff knowledgeable and experienced enough to help you get started or to assist you should you have difficulties.

Midwives (DEMs and CNMs) value the importance of immediate contact between mother and child, and promote this whenever possible. CNMs practicing in medical settings may be limited in allowing immediate bonding time based on the protocols of the neonatal doctors and nurses. Midwives with homebirth practices encourage immediate contact between mother and baby (and other family members as well), and—with the exception of neonatal emergencies—don't separate the mom and baby. Success rates with breastfeeding among their clients occurs regardless of place of birth, though midwives with homebirth practices generally have the highest rates of breastfeeding compared to all other groups.

Emergencies

Medical doctors are especially skilled at dealing with high-risk women and complications of birth. An ideal might be to see midwives attending all but the small group of women who are in this category, and to have obstetricians available for the emergency care they provide best.

Nurse-midwives working in a medical setting are also very capable of assisting high-risk women, especially when risk is based on socioeconomic factors, and they have shown excellent outcomes with such women. However, the rules which govern the practice of nurse-midwifery usually dictate that they attend only low-risk women. Nurse-midwives are trained to provide emergency care in the event of hemorrhage, immediate neonatal problems, and other complications of labor, birth, and the postpartum period. They are able to administer medications, to perform certain emergency procedures, and can assist in a cesarean. However, if an emergency arises they are required to defer care to an attending obstetrician.

Direct-entry midwives are also skilled in handling common obstetric and neonatal emergencies, and in providing emergency care until medical care is obtained, but they are limited in the medications they use, and in the emergency procedures they can perform at home. Their privileges at hospitals vary according to state legislation. Midwives have a low rate of obstetric emergencies due to careful screening, preventive care, and non-invasive care during labor, birth, and the postpartum period.

To sum up, midwifery care provides women with the greatest freedom of choice, and is most centered on the needs of women. It is well documented that this model of care is not only the most comfortable for women, but it also results in the healthiest outcomes with the fewest complications. For some women, the hospital is the most reassuring place to have a baby, but for many women, working with a midwife is a safe and satisfying way to experience pregnancy and birth.

Choosing a Midwife

FINDING A MIDWIFE

In states where midwifery is legally recognized, finding a midwife can be as simple as looking in the phone book or contacting the state department of health for a listing. In states where midwifery is not legal, the challenge can be greater—but not impossible. Speak with local childbirth educators and La Leche League leaders, ask around at health food stores, and ask other alternative health practitioners such as chiropractors, massage therapists, herbalists, and naturopathic doctors. Even a call to a doctor's office or nurse-midwifery practice can yield information about midwives. In some locations you may have to be persistent and ask a lot of questions. In Appendix 2 "National Midwifery Organizations," you will find a listing of national organizations that can provide you with information on midwives in your area.

INTERVIEWING A MIDWIFE

The first step in choosing a midwife is the initial phone call. Call several midwives and discuss your interests, needs, and the concerns you have for your pregnancy and the birth of your child. Most midwives offer a free initial consultation. You may know exactly what you are looking for in a midwife, or it may take meeting several midwives to decide what it is you want. You must feel comfortable and able to speak freely with your midwife, as well as feel confident in her skills. Her appearance and the appearance of her office may be important indicators for you, her listening skills may attract you to working with her, or you might be drawn to her philosophies of care. The following questions can help you interview midwives. Bring this list along with you and add your own questions to the list.

The Midwife Questionnaire

1. What is your training and experience? How much experience have you had with homebirth practice (or with the setting in which you practice)?

2. Why are you a midwife? What are your philosophies of care?

3. What are your expectations of me and my family regarding self-care and involvement? Do you expect my partner to be at each prenatal visit?

4. How often do we meet prenatally and what do we do at prenatal visits? How much time can I expect to have with you at each visit? What tests do you require me to have? Do you expect me to take prenatal classes?

5. Do you work alone or with assistants? What are your assistants' qualifications? Can I choose the assistant or meet the assistant before the birth? Are you affiliated with any obstetricians? Pediatricians? Other practitioners?

6. What equipment do you bring to births? Do you carry any emergency equipment such as medications for bleeding, oxygen, or other resuscitation equipment?

7. What experience have you had with complications, and what have been some of the outcomes of those situations? Do you know how to handle a hemorrhage and how to resuscitate a newborn? Are there any complications that you think I should know about?

8. How do you handle emergencies? What do we do if I need medical care? Do you have medical back-up or can you recommend physicians? Will you come to the hospital with me? What will your role be?

9. What are your fees and what do your fees cover? What, exactly, do your services include? Will there be other

expenses (such as lab work, supplies, childbirth classes)? What happens if we transfer to medical care before labor or during labor? Can you be reimbursed by insurance? Do you have a specific payment schedule?

10. How many births do you generally attend per month? Will there be another midwife available for me if you are at another birth?

11. How can I reach you in an emergency or when I am in labor (pager, answering service, etc.)?

13. When do you come to the home during labor? What do you do routinely during labor? How long do you stay after the birth? What do you expect from me during labor?

12. Do you provide postpartum care? Where? How often? What does this include? For how long am I entitled to post-partum care from you?

13. What are your policies regarding unusual situations (for example breech births, twins, or if I am overdue)?

14. How does your personal/family life impact your availability? If you have young children of your own, what are your plans for them when I go into labor? Do you ever take personal vacations? What do I do if you are away and I need a midwife?

15. Can you provide me with references of other people you have attended?

After the interview, ask yourself if you are comfortable with this person. Do you like her? Does she seem honest? Can you be honest with her? Is she warm and caring? Clean? Organized? Do her values seem compatible with yours? Do you think you would feel comfortable with her at your birth?

THE PERFECT ATTENDANT

The perfect attendant does not exist, but you can find some-one with whom you can develop a comfortable relationship. What's more important than finding the "perfect attendant" is realizing that working with a midwife—especially when planning a homebirth—is a matter of taking personal responsibility. You will need to be actively involved in your own prenatal care and education—eating well, resting, exercising, and educating yourself. No birth attendant in any environment can control the labor you have, how your birth goes, or the outcome. No birth attendant can give life or prevent death—some things are beyond human control. In recognizing this you can find someone to work with who meets your standards for care without placing unrealistic expectations on any person, setting, or philosophy, and without placing unreasonable expectations on yourself.

MEDICAL BACK-UP

Whether your midwife has medical back-up will depend upon the legality of midwifery in your community, the availability and willingness of doctors to provide medical back-up, and you midwife's philosophy of care. In states where midwifery is legal, obstetricians are more willing to provide medical back-up for midwifery clients, but in states where midwifery is not legal, doctors may be too scared about jeopardizing their practices to get involved. In some cases, physicians are willing to work out creative back-up relationships with midwives they trust, or to work with individual clients but not directly with the midwives.

COSTS

A national average of midwifery fees ranges from $800 to $3000, with rural midwives charging the lowest, and cosmopolitan midwives in legal states charging the highest fees. The average fee nationally is about $1500. Midwifery services generally include complete prenatal care, attendance during labor and birth, and anywhere from one to four postpartum visits, plus postpartum phone calls. Postpartum care generally extends for six weeks after the birth. Direct-entry midwifery care at a birthing center will often fall in the upper half of that price range, and services will be similar, though visits and birth attendance will occur at the clinic, not at your home. There will usually be additional costs for lab work, running between $75 and $200. No further testing is required unless medically indicated, but any further tests would also be at your own expense.

The cost of childbirth classes as well as supplies for your birth are your responsibility and are not included in most midwives' fees. Your midwife will generally pay for any assistants she brings to your birth unless you specifically request someone who is beyond her pay scale.

Should you require transfer to medical care prior to your birth, your midwife will prorate her fees based on services rendered. However, should you transfer to medical care during labor, in most cases, no money is returned and the costs of medical care are your responsibility.

In contrast to fees for working with a direct-entry midwife for a homebirth, the costs of working with an obstetrician for a normal vaginal birth is between $2500 and $3500, and in addition to that you must pay a facility fee of approximately $4000 or more to the hospital. For a cesarean, your provider fee (the cost for your obstetrician) will rise by as much as $3000, in addition to the facility fee. Lab tests and ultrasounds are additional costs, as are longer stays in the hospital. It is not uncommon to be told that you cannot enter an obstetric practice until you have paid a large portion of your total fee, as much as $1500 at an initial visit.

Fees for working with a nurse-midwife can range from as low as $2500 for provider and facility fee combined, to $4500 for provider and facility fee combined. Nurse midwife fees generally fall between those of direct-entry midwives and obstetricians. (These fees are based on figures from 1994–1997.)

THIRD-PARTY REIMBURSEMENT

Third-party reimbursement depends upon the laws pertaining to midwifery in your community. However, even in states where midwifery is not legally recognized, private insurance companies will sometimes provide reimbursement to the parents when they provide a receipt from the midwife or if the midwife files the insurance papers. Some midwives are willing to wait for payment from the insurance company, others would rather have you pay the fee to the midwife and have you be reimbursed by the insurance company. Many homebirth families have been able to receive full reimbursement for their expenses. You will need to pursue this matter with your midwife and your insurance company.

Medicaid rarely reimburses for midwifery expenses except in states where midwifery is legally recognized.

MALPRACTICE INSURANCE

Most direct-entry midwives are not covered by malpractice insurance, and in fact, many choose not to be in order to avoid the litigious mindset so prominent in the practice of obstetrics. That is, care providers making decisions about care based upon insurance considerations rather than the needs of those they serve. Some midwives do wish to be insured, and there are several companies now offering such coverage.

Midwifery and the Law

Presently the midwifery profession in the United States is at a crossroads. Laws from state to state are inconsistent. States as close in proximity as Massachusetts and New York can have tremendously different legal situations for midwifery practice, ranging from completely legal status without requiring licensure, to outright felony status. While midwives in Massachusetts can practice freely and openly, midwives in New York are being served cease and desist orders, are being threatened with legal action, and are being arrested, facing possible jail sentences. How is it that midwives fare so well in safety statistics and can be legal in one state, yet be considered criminals and a threat to public safety in a neighboring state? This is particularly poignant in New York where large numbers of women go without prenatal care and where low-birth weight and infant mortality rates are high compared to national and international standards. Many states are passing new legislation to allow provisions for the legal practice of midwifery, while a few states are further restricting it. To find out the current status of midwifery in your state, contact the Midwives' Alliance of North America (MANA) or the North American Registry of Midwives (NARM).

The late Jessica Mitford, in her book *The American Way of Birth*, provides several striking examples of the treatment of midwives by law enforcement agencies. She includes a case in California in the 1980s in which a midwife with an excellent reputation and a successful practice was held, along with her children, at gun point by state police while her house was searched and many of her personal and professional possessions were confiscated. Such preposterous situations are relics of ridiculous misconceptions about mid-wives that are centuries old. Nonetheless, they continue to be used to shape politics and to cause legal authorities to plague midwives. What other professional would ever be treated this way?

BIRTH IS NOT A MEDICAL EVENT

The view held by the medical profession that childbearing is an event requiring intensive medical management leads to the accusation that midwifery is the practice of medicine. Yet midwives view childbearing as a natural event that proceeds best in the absence of medical management.

According to internationally known anthropologist and childbirth educator-activist Shelia Kitzinger, "A carefully planned and lovingly conducted homebirth, in which the rhythms of nature are respected and the woman is nurtured by attendants who have the knowledge and understanding to support the spontaneous unfolding of life, is the safest kind of birth there is, and the most satisfying for everyone involved." (Kitzinger, 1991) This statement is born out in a well-designed scientific study conducted by Dr. Lewis Mehl and colleagues, when he matched 1046 women planning homebirths with the same number of women planning hospital births, and studied the outcomes. Note that all homebirth cases that required hospital transports were attributed to the homebirth group, so the hospital group does not include these cases. These were a few of the results:

- The hospital births had five times the incidence of maternal high blood pressure, possibly indicative of greater physical and emotional stress;

- The hospital births had three and one-half times the amount of meconium staining, fetal bowel movement excreted into the amniotic fluid, indicative of fetal stress;
- The hospital births had eight times the incidence of shoulder dystocia, a situation in which the fetal shoulders become stuck after the head is born;
- Infant deaths both during and after birth were essentially the same for the two groups;
- Apgar scores were better for homebirths, though these scores are subjectively determined by the care provider;
- Over three times as many babies in the hospital required resuscitation;
- Four times as many babies in the hospital became infected;
- Thirty times as many hospital babies incurred birth injuries;
- Less than 5 percent of homebirth women received analgesics while 75 percent of women in the hospital were administered drugs;
- Cesarean sections were three times higher in the hospital group;
- Nine times as many episiotomies were done in the hospital group, and nine times as many severe (third- and fourth-degree) tears occurred in the hospital group. (Mehl in Suarez, 1993).

The World Health Organization corroborated this view with a 1981 report stating that midwifery and nursing are separate disciplines, and they should be studied and considered separately (Suarez 1993). Until the cultural view of childbearing is one of respect for and trust in women's bodies, it is likely that midwives will continue to be swimming against the current in the effort to provide women with woman-centered care.

FREEDOM OF CHOICE, FREEDOM OF PROFESSION

Women should be free to choose the type of care they receive during pregnancy and birth, including care provider and setting. When midwifery is illegal, it is obviously more difficult for women to find midwives. The stigma of illegality can compromise a woman's sense of security with her care provider. At a time when a woman needs to be focusing on herself and her baby, not on legal issues, she doesn't need the added stress that can result from not seeing a legally recognized medical care practitioner. These burdens also affect the midwife, as she is constantly aware that her illegal status could have a severely negative impact on her own life and that of her family, should she ever be drawn into a legal battle or arrested.

Current legislation in many states not only impinges upon women's freedom of choice but it impinges upon the constitutional right of midwives to practice their profession. "State power is supposed to provide for the general welfare of citizens and secure them against the consequences of ignorance, deception, and fraud. Broad medical practice acts that protect unsubstantiated medical assertions and make criminals of competent midwives provides no such security" (Suarez 1993).

Furthermore, sexism comes into play in government involvement. Legislators assume that women who are choosing midwives are ignorant, rather than recognizing that women choosing midwives tend to be well-educated women making informed decisions.

THE SOCIAL BENEFITS OF
MIDWIFERY CARE

In the United States we currently have over 600 neonatal intensive care units, reflecting the serious problem we have with neonatal problems—the greatest of which is low-birth-weight babies. Yet midwifery care has been shown to substantially reduce low birthweight. Unfortunately, a large percentage of those having low-birthweight babies are those women who are considered medically indigent—those who are unlikely to receive prenatal care and education, and are likely to have poor nutrition.

We are pouring millions of dollars annually into the medical care of premature babies for this country's poor women. Yet half of these babies will still grow up with cerebral palsy, mental retardation, learning disabilities, and other serious problems, which will continue to cause individual human suffering while costing exorbitant amounts of money for special programs and public assistance.

Because of legislation and insurance company policies that do not allow for the legal practice and reimbursement of midwives, large numbers of women will continue to give birth to compromised babies. The most responsible and financially sensible approach is prevention, and this becomes highly possible with the presence of large numbers of midwives available to provide prenatal care and childbirth services. The National Commission to Prevent Infant Mortality has suggested that even minor improvements in preventative care would result in an immediate savings of 75 to 90 million dollars (Suarez 1993). However, requiring women to first obtain a nursing degree and then specialty training as a midwife for several years will significantly reduce the numbers of women desiring to, or able to, enter the profession.

A COMMON EFFORT

Making midwifery care legal would remove the shroud of tension that surrounds illegal practice, while making this highly effective option available to a broader base of women and babies. Midwives recognize the need for, and welcome the medical expertise of obstetricians, nurse-midwives, and other specialists in the care of childbearing women and their babies. Midwifery care is based on women receiving the care that is best for them, whether this be with an obstetrician in the hospital, or a woman in her own home with a midwife. While midwifery care is based on the premise that childbearing is a normal and healthy event, midwives are well aware that complications can arise necessitating emergency medical care. Therefore midwives welcome the mutual and interrelated interests of all practitioners in this area, and seek to create an environment with options that are not mutually exclusive. It is up to medical care providers to also recognize the benefits of a mutually supportive environment, both for childbearing women and for practitioners.

To find out the current status of midwifery in your state contact the Midwives' Alliance of North America (MANA) or the North American Registry of Midwives (NARM).

WHAT YOU CAN DO

Families who have received midwifery care are among the most effective vehicles for creating changes in the legal status of midwifery—consumer power is a strong force in the American economic and legal world. Nationally, consumers have been a strong force for getting midwifery more broadly accepted. Through contacting the national midwifery organizations listed in Appendix 2, you will find other people both in your community and nationally who are also committed to freedom of choice in childbearing, and who wish to make midwifery care a legally available option for all women.

The most effective changes on a state-by-state basis have come not from court battles but from legislative pressure. According to Suzanne Suarez, lawyer, midwifery advocate, and author of "Midwifery is Not the Practice of Medicine" for the *Yale Journal of Law and Feminism*, "Unless proponents can convince skeptical courts that midwifery is a fundamental constitutional right, prompting strict scrutiny of state regulations restricting its availability, activists should focus on convincing legislatures that independent...midwifery is in the best interest of the state. Proponents should present to legislators the evidence that changes in midwifery could save lives and money."

It has been well established that there are risks involved in hospital birth. It has also been shown that midwifery care and homebirth are safe options for many mothers and babies. A sense of empowerment, self-confidence, and control, as well as the opportunity for peacefully welcoming their babies into the world, is the greatest benefit that midwives impart to childbearing families.

Appendix I
CIMS Model of Maternity Care

Following are excerpts from The Mother-Friendly Childbirth Initiative:

PRINCIPLES
We believe the philosophical cornerstones of mother-friendly care to be as follows:

Normalcy of the Birthing Process
- Birth is a normal, natural, and healthy process.
- Women and babies have the inherent wisdom necessary for birth.
- Babies are aware, sensitive human beings at the time of birth, and should be acknowledged and treated as such.
- Breastfeeding provides the optimum nourishment for newborns and infants.
- Birth can safely take place in hospitals, birth centers, and homes.
- The midwifery model of care, which supports and protects the normal birth process, is the most appropriate for the majority of women during pregnancy and birth.

Empowerment
- A woman's confidence and her ability to give birth and to care for her baby are enhanced or diminished by every person who gives her care, and by the environment in which she gives birth.
- A mother and baby are distinct yet interdependent during pregnancy, birth, and infancy. Their interconnectedness is vital and must be respected.

- Pregnancy, birth, and the postpartum period are milestone events in the continuum of life. These experiences profoundly affect women, babies, fathers, and families, and have important and long-lasting effects on society.

Autonomy

Every woman should have the opportunity to:

- Have a healthy and joyous birth experience for herself and her family, regardless of her age or circumstances;

- Give birth as she wishes in an environment in which she feels nurtured and secure, and her emotional well-being, privacy, and personal preferences are respected;

- Have access to the full range of options for pregnancy, birth, and nurturing her baby, and to accurate information on all available birthing sites, caregivers, and practices;

- Receive accurate and up-to-date information about the benefits and risks of all procedures, drugs, and tests suggested for use during pregnancy, birth, and the postpartum period, with the rights to informed consent and informed refusal;

- Receive support for making informed choices about what is best for her and her baby based on her individual values and beliefs.

Do No Harm

- Interventions should not be applied routinely during pregnancy, birth, or the postpartum period. Many standard medical tests, procedures, technologies, and drugs carry risks to both mother and baby, and should be avoided in the absence of specific scientific indications for their use.

- If complications arise during pregnancy, birth, or the postpartum period, medical treatments should be evidence-based.

Responsibility

- Each caregiver is responsible to the quality of care she or he provides.

- Maternity care practice should be based not on the needs of the caregiver or provider, but solely on the needs of the mother and child.

- Each hospital and birth center is responsible for the periodic review and evaluation, according to current scientific evidence, of the effectiveness, risks, and rates of use of its medical procedures for mothers and babies.

- Society, through both its government and the public health establishment, is responsible for ensuring access to maternity services for all women, and for monitoring the quality of those services.

- Individuals are ultimately responsible for making informed choices about the health care they and their babies receive.

TEN STEPS OF THE MOTHER-FRIENDLY CHILDBIRTH INITIATIVE FOR MOTHER-FRIENDLY HOSPITALS, BIRTH CENTERS, AND HOME BIRTH SERVICES

To receive CIMS designation as "mother-friendly," a hospital, birth center, or home birth service must carry out the above philosophical principles by fulfilling the Ten Steps of Mother-Friendly Care:

A mother-friendly hospital, birth center, or home birth service:

1. Offers all birthing mothers:

   — Unrestricted access to the birth companions of her choice, including fathers, partners, children, family members, and friends;

   — Unrestricted access to continuous emotional and physical support from a skilled woman—for example a doula, or labor support professional;

   — Access to professional midwifery care.

2. Provides accurate descriptive and statistical information to the public about its practices and procedures for birth care, including measures of interventions and outcomes.

3. Provides culturally competent care—that is, care that is sensitive to the specific beliefs, values, and customs of the mother's ethnicity and religion.

4. Provides the birthing woman with the freedom to walk, move about, and assume positions of her choice during labor and birth (unless restriction is specifically required to correct a complication), and discourages the use of the lithotomy (flat on back with legs elevated) position.

5. Has clearly defined policies and procedures for:

   — collaborating and consulting throughout the perinatal period with other maternity services, including communicating with the original caregiver when transfer from one birth site to another is necessary;

   — linking the mother and baby to appropriate community resources, including prenatal and post-discharge follow-up and breastfeeding support.

6. Does not routinely employ practices and procedures that are unsupported by scientific evidence, including but not limited to the following:

   — shaving;

   — enemas;

   — IVs (intravenous drip);

   — withholding nourishment;

   — early rupture of membranes;

   — electronic fetal monitoring.

Other interventions are limited as follows:

   — An oxytocin use rate of 10% or less for induction and augmentation;

   — An episiotomy rate of 20% or less, with a goal of 5% or less;

   — A total cesarean rate of 10% or less in community hospitals, and 15% or less in tertiary care (high-risk) hospitals;

— A VBAC (vaginal birth after cesarean) rate of 60% or more, with a goal of 75% or more.

7. Educates staff in non-drug methods of pain relief, and does not promote the use of analgesic or anesthetic drugs not specifically required to correct a complication.

8. Encourages all mothers and families, including those with sick or premature newborns or infants with congenital problems, to touch, hold, breastfeed, and care for their babies to the extent compatible with their conditions.

9. Discourages non-religious circumcision of the newborn.

10. Strives to achieve the WHO-UNICEF "Ten Steps of the Baby-Friendly Hospital Initiative" to promote successful breastfeeding which are:

   — Have a written breastfeeding policy communicated to all health care staff;
   — Train all health care staff in skills necessary to implement this policy;
   — Inform all pregnant women about the benefits and management of breastfeeding;
   — Help mothers initiate breastfeeding within a half-hour of birth;
   — Show mothers how to breastfeed and how to maintain lactation even if they should be separated from their infants;
   — Give newborn infants no food or drink other than breast milk unless medically indicated;
   — Practice rooming in: allow mothers and infants to remain together 24 hours a day;
   — Encourage breastfeeding on demand;
   — Give no artificial teat or pacifiers (also called dummies or soothers) to breastfeeding infants;
   — Foster the establishment of breastfeeding support groups and refer mothers to them on discharge from hospitals or clinics.

Appendix 2
National Midwifery Organizations

The following organizations can provide you with information on midwives in your area, as well as on midwifery training, certification, and accreditation.

Midwives Alliance of North America (MANA)
PO Box 175
Newton, KS 67114
316-283-4543

North American Registry of Midwives (NARM)
1044 Woodlawn
Iowa City, IA 52245
319-354-5365

Citizens for Midwifery (CFM)
PO Box 82227
Athens, GA 30608
316-267-7236

Midwifery Education and Accreditation Council
318 W. Birch, Suite 5
Flagstaff, AZ 86001
520-214-0997

American College of Nurse-Midwives (ACNM)
818 Connecticut Avenue, NW, Suite 900
Washington, DC 20006
202-728-9860

Bibliography

Arms, Suzanne. *Immaculate Deception II: A Fresh Look at Childbirth*. Berkeley: Celestial Arts, 1994.

Baul, Mary Ann. "The Value of MEAC Accreditation." *Citizens for Midwifery News*, Vol. 2 Issue 2. (April, 1997).

Baldwin, Rahima. *Special Delivery: The Complete Guide to Informed Birth*. Berkeley: Celestial Arts: 1979.

Cairns, Ann. "Midwifery Model of Care." *MANA News*. Vol. XIV No. 3. (July, 1996).

Childbirth Alternatives Quarterly. "The U.S. is Still Declining in World Infant Mortality Ranking." *Childbirth Alternatives Quarterly*. Vol. IX, No. 2 (Winter, 1988).

Coalition for Improving Maternity Services. *The Mother-Friendly Childbirth Initiative*. Washington, DC.: CIMS c/o ASPO/LAMAZE, 1996.

Cunningham, J. D. "Experiences of Australian Mothers Who Gave Birth Either at Home, at a Birth Center, or in Hospital Labor Wards." *Social Science and Medicine*. 36(4): 475–83, February, 1993.

Davis, Elizabeth. *Heart and Hands: A Midwife's Guide to Pregnancy and Birth*. Berkeley: Celestial Arts, 1987.

Davis-Floyd, Robbie E. *Birth as an American Right of Passage*. Berkeley: University of California Press, 1992.

Durand, Mark. "The Safety of Home Birth: The Farm Study." *Journal of the American Public Health Association*. 82: 450–452. (March, 1992).

Ehrenreich, Barbara and Deidre English. *Witches, Midwives, and Nurses: A History of Woman Healers*. Old Westbury New York: Feminist Press, 1973.

Enkin, Murray, et. al. *A Guide to Effective Care in Pregnancy and Childbirth*. Oxford: Oxford University Press, 1995.

Eskes, T. K. "Home Deliveries in The Netherlands—Perinatal mortality and Morbidity."
International Journal of Gynecology and Obstetrics. 38(3): 161–9, July, 1992.

Flint, Caroline. "Should Midwives Train as Florists." *Arena*. London: United Kingdom, 1988.

Frye, Anne. *Holistic Midwifery: A Comprehensive Textbook for Midwives in Homebirth Practice*. Portland, Oregon: Labrys Press, 1995.

Gabay, Mary and Sidney Wolfe. *Unnecessary Cesarean Sections: Curing a National Epidemic*. Washington, DC: Public Citizen Publications, 1994.

Gaskin, Ina May. *Midwives: An Untapped Resource*. On-line, 1994.

___ *Spiritual Midwifery*. Summertown, Tennessee: The Book Publishing Company, 1980.

Goer, Henci. *Obstetric Myths Versus Research Realties: A Guide to the Medical Literature*. Westport, Connecticut: Bergin and Garvey, 1995.

Hafner, Eaton C. and L. K. Pearce. "Birth Choices, the Law, and Medicine: Balancing Individual Freedoms and Protection of the Public's Health." *Journal of Health Politics, Policy, and Law*. 19(4): 813–35, Winter, 1994.

Hallett, Elizabeth and Karen Ehrlich. *Midwife Means "With Woman": A Guide to Healthy Childbearing*. Sacramento, California: California Association of Midwives, 1991.

Hinds, M. Ward et. al. "Neonatal Outcome in Planned v. Unplanned Out-of-Hospital Births in Kentucky." *Journal of the American Medical Association*. Vol. 253, No. 11. (March, 1985).

Hoff, Gerard Alan and Lawrence J. Schneiderman. "Having Babies at Home: Is It Safe? Is It Ethical?" *Hastings Center Report*. Vol. 15, No. 6. (December, 1985).

Janssen, P. A. et. al. "Licensed Midwife-attended, Out-of-Hospital Births in Washington State: Are They Safe?" *Birth*. 21(3): 141–8, September 1994.

King, Kenny P., et. al. "Satisfaction with Postnatal Care—the Choice of Home or Hospital." *Midwifery*. 9(3): 146–53, September, 1993.

Kitzinger, Sheila. *Homebirth: The Essential Guide to Giving Birth Outside of the Hospital*. New York: Dorling Kindersley, 1991.

Maurath, Pam. *Legal Status of Direct Entry midwives: State by State Analysis*. Midwives Alliance of North America, Midwifery Education and Accreditation Council, and the North American Registry of Midwives. May, 1997.

Mehl, Lewis, et. al. "Outcomes of Elective Home Births: A Series of 1,146 Cases." *Journal of Reproductive Medicine*. Vol. 19, No. 5. (November, 1977).

Midwives' Alliance of New York. *Midwives Caring for New York's Women*. Warwick, New York, March 1, 1990.

Midwives' Alliance of North America Position Statements. "Access to Midwifery Care."

___ "Statement of Values and Ethics"

___ "Core Competencies for Midwifery Practice." (1997).

___ "Standards and Qualifications for the Art and Practice of Midwifery." (January, 1997).

Midwives' Alliance of North America Fact Sheets. "The Safety of Homebirth." (1997).

___ "Cesarean Section in the U.S." (1997).

___ "Midwife-Attended Birth." (1997).

___ "Midwife Facts." (1997).

___ "Maternity Care: An International Perspective." (1997).

Mitford, Jessica. *The American Way of Birth*. New York: Dutton, 1992.

Mothering Magazine. "Midwife Deliveries on the Increase." *Mothering Magazine*. Summer, 1997.

Mothering Magazine. "Mothering Perinatal Healthcare Index." *Mothering Magazine*. Fall, 1993.

Olsen, O. "Home Delivery and Scientific Reasoning." [Norwegian] *Source Tidsskrift for Den Norske Laegeforening*. 114(30): 3655–7, December 10, 1994.

Poole, Catherine and Elizabeth Parr. *Choosing a Nurse Midwife*. New York: John Wiley and Sons, 1994.

Rothman, Barbara Katz. *The Encyclopedia of Childbearing*. New York: Henry Holt, 1993.

___ *In Labor: Women and Power in the Birthplace*. New York: Norton and Company, 1991.

Sakala, Carol. "Midwifery Care and Out-of-Hospital Settings: How do they Reduce Unnecessary Cesarean Section births?" *Social Science and Medicine*. 37(10): 1233–50, November, 1993.

Sears, William and Martha. *The Birth Book*. Boston: Little, Brown, and Company, 1994.

Sonnenstuhl, Pat. "Introduction to Midwifery." *Sci-Med Midwifery FAQ*. June 10, 1995.

Suarez, Suzanne. "Midwifery is Not the Practice of Medicine." *Yale Journal of Law and Feminism*. Vol. 5, No. 2 (Spring 1993).

Tew, Marjorie. "Do Obstetric Intranatal Interventions Make Birth Safer?" *British Journal of Obstetrics and Gynecology*. Vol. 93, 659–674. (July, 1986).

___ "We Have the Technology." *Nursing Times*, November 20, 1985.

Tyson, H. "Outcomes of 1001 Midwife-attended Home Births in Toronto, 1983–1988." *Birth*. 18(1): 14–9, March, 1991.

Ubell, Earl. "Are Births As Safe As They Could Be?" *Parade Magazine*. February 7, 1993.

Wagner, Marsden. "A Global Witch-hunt." *Lancet* 1995; 346: 1020–22.

___ "Active Management of Labor." April, 1995.

___ "Pursuing the Birth Machine: The Search for Appropriate Birth Technology. Camperdown, Australia: ACE Graphics, 1994.

___ "Is Homebirth Dangerous?" *The Birth Gazette*. Vol. 5, No. 4 (Fall, 1989).

___ "Testimony Before the US Commission to Prevent Infant Mortality." *Birth Gazette*. Vol. 4, No. 3. (Spring, 1988).

Willis, Sher, Nan Koehler Solomon, and Nancy Duncan. "The Traditional Midwife." *Midwifery Today*, Number 19, Autumn 1991.

Women's Institute for Childbearing Policy. *Childbearing Policy Within a National Health Program: An Evolving Consensus for New Directions*. Roxbury, Vermont: WICP, 1994.

Woodcock, H. C. et. al. "A Matched Cohort Study of Planned Home and Hospital Births in Western Australia 1981–1987." *Midwifery*. 10 (3): 125–35, September 1994.